AZHAGU MADHAVAN SIVALINGAM
GANESAN SIVAMANI
ARJUN PANDIAN

INTRODUCTION TO DIABETES MELLITUS

AZHAGU MADHAVAN SIVALINGAM
GANESAN SIVAMANI
ARJUN PANDIAN

INTRODUCTION TO DIABETES MELLITUS

DIABETES, CAUSES, PANCREATIC ISLET TRANSPLANTATION, GENETICS, SIGNS AND SYMPTOMS, COMPLICATIONS, TESTS AND DIAGNOSIS

Scholars' Press

Publisher:
Scholars' Press
is a trademark of
International Book Market Service Ltd., member of OmniScriptum Publishing Group
17 Meldrum Street, Beau Bassin 71504, Mauritius

Printed at: see last page
ISBN: 978-613-8-92491-3

INTRODUCTION TO DIABETES MELLITUS

Mr. AZHAGU MADHAVAN SIVALINGAM, M.Sc., PGDCA., PGDBI., Ph.D.,
Research scholar,
PG & Research Department of Zoology and Biotechnology,
A.V.V.M. Sri Pushpam College (Autonomous),
Poondi –613503, Thanjavur District
Tamil Nadu, India.

Dr. GANESAN SIVAMANI, M.Sc., M.Phil., Ph.D., PGDMLT., PGDCA.,
Assistant Professor
PG & Research Department of Zoology and Biotechnology
A.V.V.M. Sri Pushpam College (Autonomous)
Poondi - 613503, Thanjavur District
Tamil Nadu, India.
E-mail: ganesanmolbio@gmail.com

Dr. ARJUN PANDIAN
Assistant Professor
Department of Biotechnology
PRIST Deemed University
Thanjavur- 613403, Tamil Nadu, India.
E-mail: arjungri@gmail.com

PREFACE

This book Introduction on Diabetes Mellitus provides a concise coverage of the concepts related to diabetes in terms of different types of diabetes, causes, signs and symptoms, tests and diagnosis, complications, prevention and treatment. Health is a positive concept emphasizing social and personal resources as well as physical capabilities. Disease is a term describing any deviation from the normal state of health or wellness. It includes physical, mental and social conditions. Both health and disease are coeval with life. Since archaic time, human are interested in trying to control diseases. Medical are involved in various ways to cure human disease and control the disorders in order to bring relief to the sick.

In order to create awareness and to provide ample information to human society, this book has been designed carefully with the recent available modern tests to diagnose the disease, advanced methods to treat the complications covering all treatment and therapies such as dietary management, yoga, meditation, acupressure, acupuncture, massage therapy, aroma therapy, music therapy, biofeedback, ayurvedic herbal medicine, homeopathy and allopathic medicine.

I have ventured to write this book and hope the readers will find it very informative and enjoyable to read.

The success of any work is never limited to the individual who is dedicated for the work. Most often, it is a collective effort of friends that reflect in the success. I take this opportunity to thank my **friends** and **family** members for the completion of work.

First and foremost, I would like to express deep sense of gratitude to the **Secretary** and **Correspondent** and **Principal** of A.V.V.M. Sri Pushpam College (Autonomous), Poondi, Thanjavur (Dt.) for their encouragement the freedom of work contributed immensely to give suggestion and motivation to complete my work successfully.

We would like to express gratitude to our friends and motivated **Professors** for their kind help during manual preparation in better way.

We are immensely thankful to Iyal Publication, Thanjavur for neatly printing the Manual. Last but not the least I thank God who gave me strength and patience to do my work successfully.

Mr. S. Azhagu Madhavan

Dr. S. Ganesan

Dr. P. Arjun

Mrs. Meenambigai Ganesan

2

Dedicated our parents and our family members

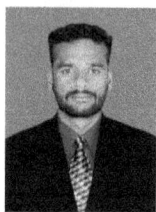

Mr. S. AZHAGU MADHAVAN, Research scholar, He has completed M.Sc., and Ph.D., Zoology from PG & Research Department of Zoology and Biotechnology, A.V.V.M. Sri Pushpam College (Autonomous), Poondi, Thanjavur Dt., Tamilnadu, India. **Mr. S. Azhagu Madhavan,** Research group is involved in studying Cell and Molecular signatures with special reference to Bioinformatics & Statistical tools Software knowledge, Mendeley, SPSS, NCBI, Origin pro-8 & Gene & Protein Sequence, Multiple Sequence Analysis, Pathway Analysis, DAVID -Bioinformatics resources & Tools, Molecular Docking Diabetes Mellitus. Our research integrates physiological and pharmacological techniques to study mechanisms underlying development and progressions of Cancer. He has presented 39 papers in National and International conference, lecture workshop and National seminar published 17 Research paper in well-reputed journals.

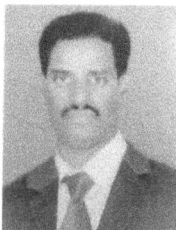

Dr. S. GANESAN, Assistant Professor, Department of Zoology and Biotechnology, A.V.V.M. Sri Pushpam College (Autonomous), Poondi, Thanjavur. He has completed M.Sc., Zoology from Madurai Kamaraj University, Madurai, M.Phil., Zoology from the University of Madras, Chennai and Ph.D., from Bharathiar University, Coimbatore. He has 12 years of experience in Research and 7 years of experience in teaching. He is a Life time member of Indian Science Congress Association, Kolkata, Member Review Board of Cancer Biology and Treatment, the USA and Life member in Association for the promotion of DNA fingerprinting & other DNA technologies. Dr Ganesan's Research group is involved in studying cell and molecular signatures with special reference to insulin secretion, insulin action and Oncological research. Our research integrates physiological and pharmacological approaches with Biochemical, Molecular Biological and Proteomics techniques to study mechanisms underlying development and progression of Diabetes, its complications and Oncological Research studies. He has submitted nearly 20 16s r DNA and Protein sequencing at NCBI, USA. He has presented 72 papers in National and International conferences and published 47 Research papers in well-reputed journals. He has guided many M.Sc., M. Phil., and Ph.D., students.

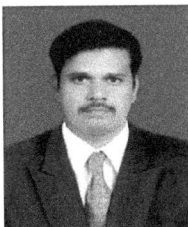

Dr. P. ARJUN, Assistant Professor, Biotechnology, PRIST Deemed University, Thanjavur. Ph.D from Centre for Advanced Studies in Botany, University of Madras, Chennai. He has 11 years of experience in teaching and Research. As a Principal Investigator currently running a three years major DBT, Goverment of India, project worth 45.69 Lakhs which is two Institute modes project (PRIST Deemed University & Gandhigram Rural University, Dindigul). Worked as a Post Doctoral Fellow for three years at Tshwane University of Technology, South Africa, two years Pharmaceutical Science (Natural Product Research), one year Crop Science (Natural Product Research). Received awards; National Research Foundation (NRF) Freestanding Post-Doctoral Fellowship for three years at South Africa and University Grants Commission (UGC) JRF Science for Meritorious Fellowship for two years at Centre for Advance Studies in Botany, has supervisor, co-supervisor and mentor various level degree courses and guiding B.Tech., B. Pharm., M. Tech., M. Pharm., M.Sc., M. Phil., D. Tech., and Ph.D. Member in professional societies; Society for Ethnopharmacology, reviewer in Journal of Ethnopharmacology, Industrial Crops and Products, HortScience, Journal of Threatened Taxa, published 38 articles in well reputed journals, book chapters, full length proceedings, presented papers international and national conference/symposium/seminars, area of specialization; Plant Biotechnology, Natural Product Research, Biological studies, Food Technology, Micro and Molecular Biology.

CONTENTS

PREFACE

INTRODUCTION

Diabetes was referred to humanity as the "Madhumeha" of classical times. This was known to Indian Ayurveda for around 3000 years as an illness with some different people whose pee was sweet enough to pull in bugs and flies. This can be found in restorative messages, for example, Charaka samhita and Sushruta samhita (400 BC). It was 'Sushruta' the incomparable Indian doctor, who analyzed during 1000 BC.

Diabetes is once viewed as a solitary ailment substance. In any case, presently it is viewed as a heterogeneous gathering of the illness described by a condition of ceaseless hyperglycemia, coming about because of a decent variety of etiologies, condition and hereditary variables, as indicated by WHO 1980. This is a long haul illness with variable clinical indications and prompts a few inconveniences like cardiovascular, renal, neurological, visual and other between current diseases.

Diabetes is an "ice sheet sickness". As indicated by ongoing assessments, the commonness of diabetes in grown-ups was around 4% worldwide and this implies more than 143 million people are currently influenced. It is anticipated that the illness pervasiveness will be 5.4% continuously 2025, with a worldwide diabetic populace arriving at 300 million.

This was portrayed over 200 years prior. It is the state of the body framework highlighted by an unreasonable release of pee with an expansion in glucose level, brought about by the debilitated emission of insulin in the body. Future might be split by this illness.

Diabetes, an interminable illness once thought to be exceptional in the creating nations, has now risen as a significant general medical issue particularly in Asian nations. An expected 30 million individuals in the southeast Asian locale are influenced. It is assessed that by 2025, there'll be almost 80 million diabetics during this district, the absolute best among all the WHO areas. In this way the South East Asian district will bear the most extreme worldwide weight of the infection.

Diabetes mellitus may be a social event of metabolic contaminations depicted by hyperglycemia achieved by insulin release, insulin movement, or both. Interminable diabetes hyperglycemia has been represented to cause longterm hurt, brokenness, and frustration of various organs, particularly the eyes, kidneys, nerves, heart, and veins.

1. HISTORY OF DIABETES

"Diabetes" springs from the Greek word sense "siphon". The Chinese name for diabetes is "sugar pee malady" which shows the sweet pee indication. This name has likewise been obtained into Korean and Japanese.

1500 BCE (Before the Common Era) - Indian doctors named the ailment as madhumeha or nectar pee which implies that the pee would draw in creepy crawlies.

400-500 CE - Indian specialists Sushruta and Charaka recognized sort 1 and type 2 diabetes as discrete conditions in which type 1 is connected with youth and type 2 with weight.

Late 1600s-The expression "Mellitus" or "from nectar" was used by Thomas Willis to segregate the condition from "diabetes insipidus" which is additionally associated with visit pee.

1776 - Matthew Dobson affirmed that the sweet taste originates from an in excess of a kind of sugar inside the pee and blood.

1869 – The Islets of Langerhans was found by an anatomist Paul Langerhans. He distinguished the keys cells inside the pancreas which produce the most substance that controls glucose levels inside the body.

(1882–1975) - specialist Charles Pybus Islet transplantation has as of late got extensive enthusiasm as a conceivably complete treatment for diabetes.

1889 - Joseph Von Mering and Oskar Minkowski found the situation of the pancreas inside-diabetes.

They found that pooches whose pancreas had been evacuated had all signs and side effects of diabetes and kicked the bucket presently.

1910 - Sir Edward Albert Sharpey-Schafer found that diabetes came about because of an absence of insulin. The term insulin is gotten from the Latin 'insula', signifying 'island'.

The 1920s-Banting and Best's Insulin Discovery in Early Revolved Diabetes Treatment and incredibly improved the forecast for what had recently been a quickly deadly illness.

1921 - Sir Frederick Grant Banting and Charles Herbert Best regular in crafted by Von Mering and Minkowski. They showed and turned around instigated diabetes in hounds by giving them a concentrate from the pancreatic islets of Langerhans of solid mutts.

1922 – Banting, Best and Collip Insulin were first effectively utilized in quite a while in decontaminated the insulin hormone from cow-like pancreas at the University of Toronto and the insulin infusions were given to the patients.

1923 – Eli Lilly and Company started the large scale manufacturing of insulin and the patients were treated in Canada and the United States.

1936 - Sir Harold Percival (Harry) Himsworth referenced the qualification between type 1 and type 2 diabetes.

November 14 – Banting's birthday was pronounced as "World Diabetes Day".

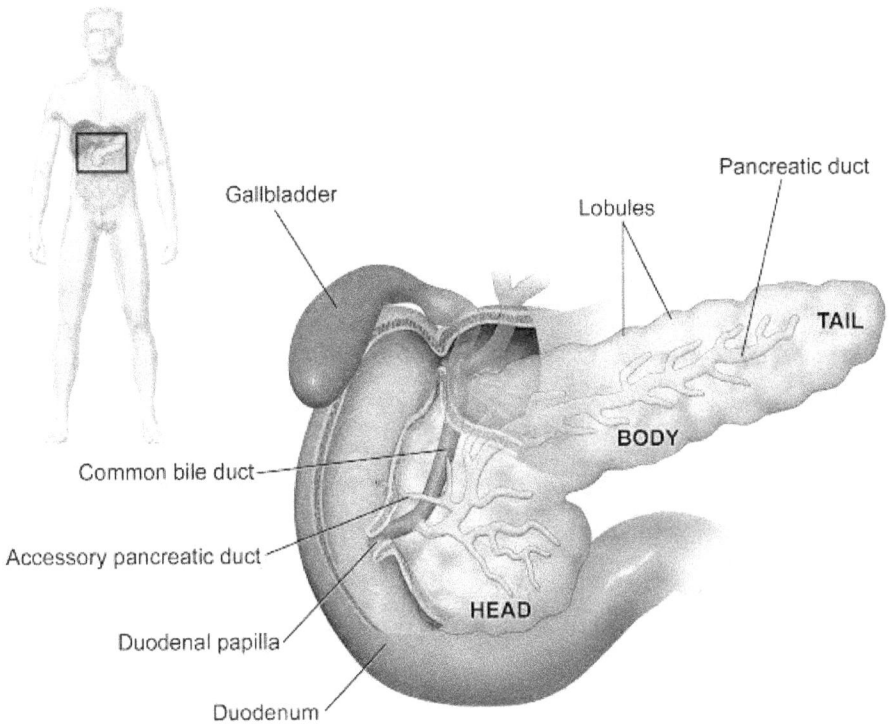

Gallbladder · Lobules · Pancreatic duct · TAIL · BODY · Common bile duct · Accessory pancreatic duct · Duodenal papilla · Duodenum · HEAD

2. DIABETES

- ✓ *Diabetes Insipidus*
  - ❖ *Cental*
  - ❖ *Nephrogenic*
  - ❖ *Dipsogenic*
  - ❖ *Gestational*
- ✓ *Diabetes Mellitus*
  - ❖ *Insulin Dependent*
  - ❖ *Non-Insulin Dependent*
  - ❖ *Gestational*
- ✓ *Bronze Diabetes*

Despite the fact that they have a typical name, diabetes mellitus and diabetes insipidus are two totally separate conditions with disconnected systems. Both reason a lot of pee to be created (polyuria). WHO (1985) classifies diabetes into two namely, Diabetes insipidus and Diabetes mellitus.

What is pre-diabetes?

Pre-diabetes is the point at which the measure of glucose in your blood is better than average yet not sufficiently high to be called diabetes. With pre-diabetes, your chances of getting type 2 diabetes, coronary sickness and stroke are higher. With some weight reduction and moderate physical action, you can postpone or forestall type 2 diabetes. You can even come back to ordinary glucose levels, perhaps without taking any meds.

Signs and manifestations of diabetes:

The signs and manifestations of diabetes are being extremely parched

- ✓ peeing frequently
- ✓ feeling hungry
- ✓ feeling tired
- ✓ getting thinner easily
- ✓ wounds that recuperate gradually
- ✓ dry, bothersome skin
- ✓ sentiments of a tingling sensation in your feet
- ✓ losing feeling in your feet
- ✓ hazy visual perception

A few people with diabetes don't have any of these signs or manifestations. The best way to know whether you have diabetes is to have your primary care physician do a blood test.

DIABETES INSIPIDUS:

Diabetes Insipidus (DI) is a condition portrayed by over the top thirst and discharge of a lot of seriously weaken pee, with a decrease of liquid admission not influence the convergence of the pee. There are various sorts.

Central Diabetes Insipidus (CDI) – Neurological form. It is the most common type in humans which involves a deficiency of antidiuretic hormone (ADH) called Arginine Vasopressin (AVP).

(1) ***Nephrogenic Diabetes Insipidus (NDI)*** – It is due to kidney or nephron dysfunction caused by an insensitivity of the kidneys or nephrons to antidiuretic hormone (ADH).

(2) ***Dipsogenic Diabetes Insipidus (DDI)*** – It is caused due to a defect or damage to the thirst mechanism located in the hypothalamus or due to mental illness. It is also known as primary polydipsia (increased thirst).

(3) ***Gestational Diabetes Insipidus (GDI)*** – It occurs only during pregnancy and the postpartum period. During pregnancy, women produce vasopressinase in the placenta, which breaks down the anti-diuretic hormone.

DIABETES MELLITUS:

In Greek, "dia" means "through", "betes" connotes "to pass" and "Mellitus" implies "sweet".

Nowadays, *Diabetes Mellitus (DM) is commonly referred to as **Diabetes**.*

✓ It is a disorder of carbohydrate metabolism which is resulting from inadequate production of insulin by the pancreas. It is characterized by the presence of sugar in the urine and excessive production of urine. It is an incessant, long lasting condition that influences your body's powerlessness to utilize the vitality found in nourishment. It is a metabolic disorder in which the body cannot properly store and use the energy found in food.

✓ Diabetes is anticipated to either the pancreas now not creating enough insulin or the cells of the body now not reacting accurately to the insulin delivered.

PANCREAS

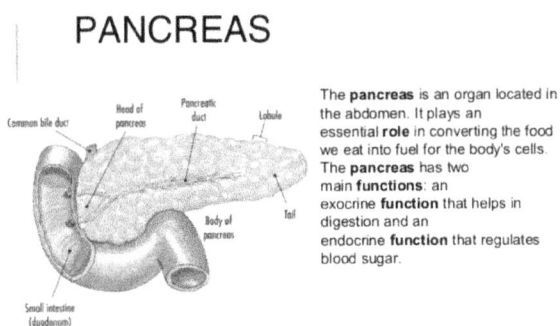

The **pancreas** is an organ located in the abdomen. It plays an essential **role** in converting the food we eat into fuel for the body's cells. The **pancreas** has two main **functions**: an exocrine **function** that helps in digestion and an endocrine **function** that regulates blood sugar.

Pancreas organ, situated between your stomach and spine, that assists with assimilation discharges a hormone it makes, called insulin, into your blood. Insulin enables your blood to convey glucose to all your body's cells. Here and there your body doesn't make enough insulin or the insulin doesn't work the manner in which it should. Glucose at that point remains in your blood and doesn't arrive at your cells. Your blood glucose levels get excessively high and can cause diabetes or prediabetes.

After some time, having a great deal of glucose in your blood can wreck prosperity.

✓ **Alpha cells:** - composing about 20% of pancreatic islet cells, it secretes glucagon which raises blood glucose level.

✓ **Beta cells:** - These secretes insulin which reduces the blood glucose level, constitute about 70% pancreatic islet cells.

✓ **Delta cells:** - constitute the 5% of pancreatic islets cells, these secrete somatostatin which provides local inhibitory regulation of insulin and glucagon release within the islet.

✓ **F cells:** - constitute the remainder of pancreatic islet cells, it secretes pancreatic polypeptide, which inhibits the secretion of somatostatin and pancreatic digestive enzyme.

There are three main types of diabetes mellitus. They are

(1) *Type 1 DM* – It is due to the failure of the pancreas to produce enough insulin. Previously it was known as *Insulin Dependent Diabetes Mellitus (IDDM)* or *Juvenile Diabetes.*

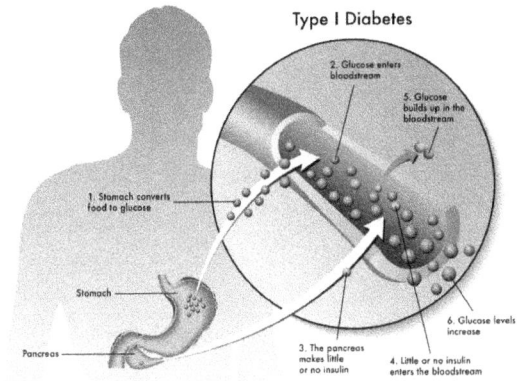

Type I Diabetes

2. Glucose enters bloodstream

5. Glucose builds up in the bloodstream

1. Stomach converts food to glucose

Stomach

Pancreas

3. The pancreas makes little or no insulin

4. Little or no insulin enters the bloodstream

6. Glucose levels increase

(2) *Type 2 DM* – It is a condition in which cells fail to respond to insulin properly. As the illness advances an absence of insulin may well similarly create. Previously it was known as *Non-Insulin Dependent Diabetes Mellitus (NIDDM)* or *Insulin Independent Diabetes Mellitus* or *Adult-Onset Diabetes.*

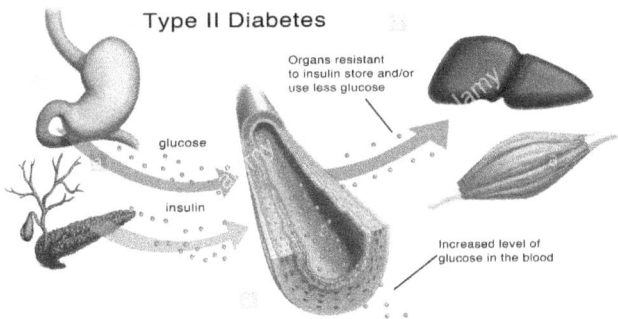

Type II Diabetes

Organs resistant to insulin store and/or use less glucose

glucose

insulin

Increased level of glucose in the blood

(3) *Gestational Diabetes* – It occurs during pregnancy without a previous history of diabetes develop a high blood sugar level. They have an increased risk of developing type 2 diabetes after pregnancy.

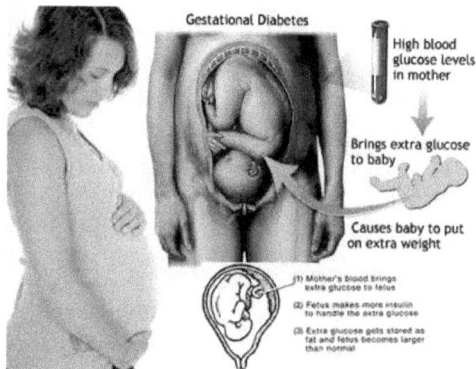

Gestational Diabetes

High blood glucose levels in mother

Brings extra glucose to baby

Causes baby to put on extra weight

(1) Mother's blood brings extra glucose to fetus

(2) Fetus makes more insulin to handle the extra glucose

(3) Extra glucose gets stored as fat and fetus becomes larger than normal

DIFFERENCES BETWEEN TYPE 1 AND TYPE 2 DIABETES:

TYPE 1 DIABETES	TYPE 2 DIABETES
Often diagnosed in childhood.	Usually diagnosed in adulthood (over 30 years old)
Not associated with excess body weight.	Often associated with excess body weight.
Often associated with higher ketone levels than the normal levels at diagnosis.	Often associated with high blood pressure (BP) and/or cholesterol levels at diagnosis.
Treated with insulin injections or insulin pumps.	Treated initially without medication or with tablets.
It cannot be controlled without taking insulin.	Sometimes possible to come out of diabetes medication.

BRONZE DIABETES:

Hemochromatosis is here and there known as bronze diabetes. Hemochromatosis is a condition where the body retains abundance iron from nourishment. The condition is brought about by a defective quality and can prompt slow harm to a few organs. The reason for this isn't known. It can prompt obscuring of the skin and hyperglycemia. This might be related with hepatic cirrhosis (a condition wherein the liver doesn't work appropriately because of long haul harm) and fibrosis (development of overabundance sinewy connective tissue in an organ or tissue) of the pancreas.

18

The symptoms are

- ➤ ardiomyopathy – debilitating of the heart
- ➤ Erectile brokenness
- ➤ Fatigue
- ➤ Increased pee
- ➤ Joint torment
- ➤ Loss of body hair
- ➤ Missed periods
- ➤ Thirst
- ➤ Unexplained bronzing or tanning of the skin

Causes:

Hemochromatosis is a generally regular acquired hereditary condition. Individuals with hemochromatosis have two arrangements of a transformed HFE quality. Individuals with one lot of the defective quality won't have hemochromatosis however could pass it on youngsters if their accomplice is additionally a bearer of the broken quality. The defective quality makes the body ingest a lot of iron from nourishment. As a rule, the body retains just as much as it needs.

The body has no normal reaction to help discharge the overabundance iron thus, throughout the years, the body stores the iron in organs, for example, the liver, pancreas and the skin, in a specific order. Overabundance iron in the liver can cause liver harm and abundance iron in the pancreas can prompt diabetes. Types of diabetes that are brought about by another ailment are alluded to as optional diabetes.

Diagnosis:

Hemochromatosis can be determined to have a transferrin immersion or serum ferritin blood test, or if necessary a DNA blood test to check for the nearness of a defective HFE quality. A liver biopsy might be completed to evaluate whether liver harm has happened. In the event that any of your nearby relatives are determined to have hemochromatosis, at that point you may wish to test for it.

Diabetes mellitus is portrayed by intermittent or industrious hyperglycemia, and is analyzed by exhibiting any of the accompanying:

✓ Fasting plasma glucose level ≥ 7.0 mmol/l (126 mg/dl)
✓ Plasma glucose ≥ 11.1 mmol/l (200 mg/dl) two hours after a 75 g oral
✓ glucose load as in a glucose resistance test
✓ Symptoms of hyperglycemia and easygoing plasma glucose ≥ 11.1 mmol/l (200 mg/dl)
✓ Glycated hemoglobin (Hb A1C) ≥ 6.5%.

A positive result, without unequivocal hyperglycemia, should be attested by a repeat of any of the above methods on a substitute day. It is desirable over measure a fasting glucose level on account of the simplicity of estimation and the extensive time responsibility of formal glucose resilience testing, which takes two hours to finish and offers negative prognostic fragment of flexibility over the fasting test. As per the present definition, two fasting glucose estimations over 126 mg/dl (7.0 mmol/l) is viewed as symptomatic for diabetes mellitus.

The World Health Organization individuals with fasting glucose levels from 6.1 to 6.9 mmol/l (110 to 125 mg/dl) are considered to have hindered fasting glucose. Individuals with plasma glucose at or above 7.8 mmol/l (140 mg/dl), however not over 11.1 mmol/l (200 mg/dl), two hours after a 75 g oral glucose load are considered to have impeded glucose resistance. Of these two prediabetic states, the last specifically is a significant hazard factor for movement to out and out diabetes mellitus, just as cardiovascular malady.

Diagnostic Criteria for Diabetes Mellitus		
Test	Cutoff	Comments
A1C *	≥6.5 %	--
Fasting plasma glucose *	≥126 mg/dL (7.0 mmol/L)	No caloric intake for > 8 hours
2-hour plasma glucose *	≥200 mg/dL (11.1 mmol/L)	After 75 g glucose in water
Random plasma glucose	≥200 mg/dL (11.1 mmol/L)	In a patient with symptoms of hyperglycemia
*A positive test requires confirmation		

Treatment:

Hemochromatosis is typically treated with customary phlebotomy, a system that includes expelling iron-rich blood from the body. An elective treatment is chelation treatment which includes taking a prescription called Deferasirox.

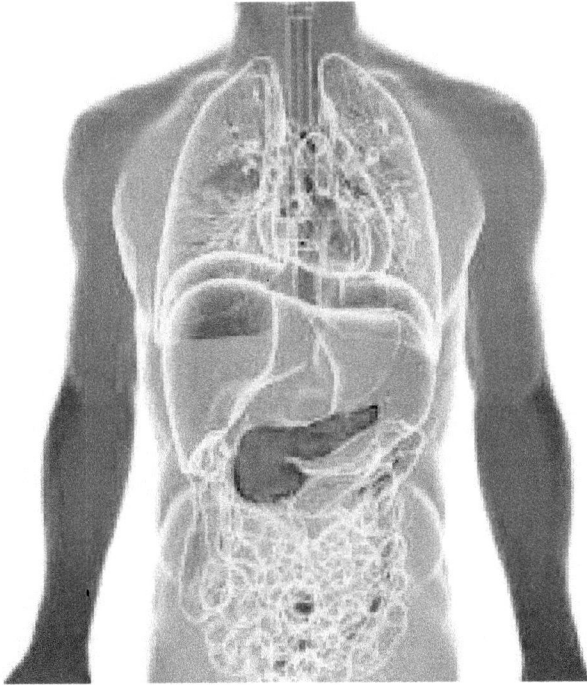

3. CAUSES OF DIABETES

The main causes of diabetes are due to

- *Pancreatic diseases*

Any illness influencing the pancreas will by implication offer ascent to diabetes. The basic malady/issue of the pancreas are as per the following:

- ✓ Any disease in pancreas
- ✓ Tumor identified with pancreas
- ✓ Removal of the pancreas by activity

Such people require insulin infusions for treatment while some may react to oral prescriptions.

Malnutrition

Diabetes in youthfulness and adulthood is created because of an absence of protein-rich nourishment in the beginning periods. Because of this, they are undernourished and extremely lean. They have next to no creation of insulin. Because of the absence of nourishment, the insulin created is inhumane and can't act appropriately. These people create diabetes gradually and react just to fake insulin.

Other hormones

In certain people, diabetes is caused because of extreme creation of specific hormones (development hormone, thyroid hormone) which meddle with the typical capacity of insulin. Because of the obstruction of such hormones, insulin neglects to do its typical exercises on nourishments and patients grow high blood glucose level which prompts diabetes.

Medicines and lethal synthetic concoctions

Certain meds, dangerous nourishment substances and synthetic concoctions wreck the insulin-delivering pancreatic cells and offers ascend to diabetes.

Liver illnesses

Certain diseases, harm and other metabolic issue identified with liver outcomes in diabetes.

Different components adding to the advancement of Diabetes:

22

Diabetes is an infection, which is because of numerous components identified with the individual and the earth and includes numerous frameworks of the body. Subsequently it is a multi-factorial and multi-framework illness. The different variables that add to the improvement of diabetes are as per the following:

Age:

Expanded age is a factor that gives more plausibility than at a more youthful age. This malady may happen at any age, yet 80% of cases happen following 50 years, frequency increment with the age factor. Diabetes may happen at any age independent of the sort. Be that as it may, most of cases are found in moderately aged and more established people. Type 1 and unhealthiness related diabetes happen in more youthful age gatherings. Later the inconveniences and treatment become unfavorable and troublesome; the result is once in a while lethal. A few specialists have likewise pronounced maturing as a significant factor for diabetes and decrepit changes in the pancreas could likewise be contributory.

Sex:

Diabetes is similarly dispersed in both the genders. Male diabetics are more in certain nations while females are more in others.

Diet and Nutrition:

In large people, type 2 diabetes was normal. Research has demonstrated that diabetes may happen regardless of nourishing status. A few investigations have indicated that kids who are given dairy animals' milk right off the bat in outset may create type 1 diabetes. This is because of the nearness of "Ox-like Serum Albumin", a substance which may harm the insulin-creating cells in the pancreas. Unreasonable starches, particularly refined sugars may by implication lead to type 2 diabetes by offering ascend to weight.

Heredity or acquire attributes:

It is because of the death of qualities starting with one age then onto the next, an individual can acquire diabetes. It relies on the closeness of blood relationship as a mother is diabetic, the hazard is 2 to 3% father is diabetic, at that point the hazard is more than the past case and if both the guardians are diabetic, the youngster has a higher hazard for diabetes.

Poor diet (lack of healthy sustenance related diabetes):

Inappropriate nourishment, low protein and fiber consumption, the high vitality admission of refined items are the normal explanations behind creating diabetes mellitus.

Obesity and fat conveyance:

Being overweight demonstrates expanded insulin obstruction that is if muscle to fat ratio over 30%, BMI 25+, midriff grith 35 creeps in ladies or 40 crawls in guys.

Stress:

Either physical damage or enthusiastic aggravation is oftentimes accused as the underlying reason for the diabetic. Any unsettling influence in corticosteroid or ACTH treatment may prompt clinical indications of diabetes.

Drug-prompted:

Clozapine (Clozaril), olanzapine (Zyprexa), risperidone (Risperdal), quetiapine (Seroquel) and ziprasidone (Geodon) are known to prompt this deadly illness.

Infection:

A portion of the staphylococci should be a capable factor for contamination in the pancreas.

Gender:

Diabetes is normally found in senior people especially guys in any case, unequivocally in ladies and those females with various pregnancies or experiencing (PCOS) polycystic ovarian disorder.

Hypertension:

Hypertension had been accounted for in numerous investigations that there is an immediate connection between high systolic weight and diabetes.

Lifestyle:

The way of life of people can end up being a hazard factor for creating diabetes.

Sedentary Lifestyle:

Individuals with an increasingly inactive way of life are inclined to diabetes when contrasted with the individuals who practice thrice seven days, are at generally safe of falling prey to diabetes.

The absence of activity adjusts the activity of insulin and its receptors.

Urbanized Lifestyle:

Factual assessment of the predominance of diabetes in created versus creating nations and country versus urban populaces have indicated fascinating discoveries. Individuals relocating from creating to created or country to urban regions show an expansion in the predominant pace of diabetes.

In this manner urbanized or westernized way of life advances the improvement of diabetes.

Psychological factors:

Mental pressure, tension, discouragement and other mental sicknesses can encourage diabetes. The pressure of any sort can cause diabetes in defenseless people. Stress might be as medical procedure, contaminations, damage, pregnancy or mental strain because of various reasons.

Heredity and different components:

Diabetes might be acquired from guardians, grandparents and blood family members. Expanded sexual movement, constant infections like Tuberculosis (TB), heaps, venereal illnesses, and so on can offer ascent to diabetes.

The beneath organization includes about the different elements associated with the advancement of Type 1 and 2 Diabetes:

FEATURES	DIABETES TYPE 1	DIABETES TYPE 2
Cause	Beta cells in the pancreas are assaulted by the body's resistant framework, in this way lessening insulin creation, prompting raised blood glucose. Insulin isn't created or is delivered in inadequate amounts.	Persistently high admissions of dietary sugars lead to overabundance requests on insulin generation, which prompts insulin obstruction after some time. Receptor cells that have gotten less touchy (impervious) to insulin can't expel glucose from the blood, prompting higher blood glucose and more noteworthy requests on insulin generation.
Genetic basis	Hereditary basis Possibly. Much of the time of type 1 diabetes, the patient would need to acquire hazard factors from both parents. Type 2 diabetes has a more grounded connection to family ancestry and heredity than type 1.	Substantial effects Thought to be activated via immune system demolition of the beta cells. The immune system assault may happen following a viral contamination, for example, mumps, rubella, cytomegalovirus.
Bodily effects	Substantial impacts Thought to be activated via immune system demolition of the beta cells. The autoimmune attack may occur following a viral infection such as mumps, rubella, cytomegalovirus.	Has all the earmarks of being identified with maturing, inert way of life, diet, hereditary impact and stoutness.
Diet	Diet Early diet may likewise assume a job. Type 1 diabetes is less basic in individuals who were breastfed and in the individuals who previously ate strong nourishments at later ages.	Obesity will in general run in families, and families will in general have comparable eating and exercise propensities. Diets high in basic sugars and low in fiber and indispensable supplements are bound to prompt diabetes.

4. PANCREATIC ISLET TRANSPLANTATION

Pancreatic Islet Transplantation, Treatment for, donor and recipient the prognosis of type-1 diabetes mellitus (T1DM) has progressed dramatically during the last century, but the disease remains a major cause of morbidity and mortality.

History of Islet Transplantation

Islet transplantation has as of late got significant enthusiasm as a conceivably authoritative treatmen for diabetes. The idea of islet transplantation isn't new agents as right on time as the Englis specialist Charles Pybus (1882–1975 endeavored to unite pancreatic tissue to fix diabetes.

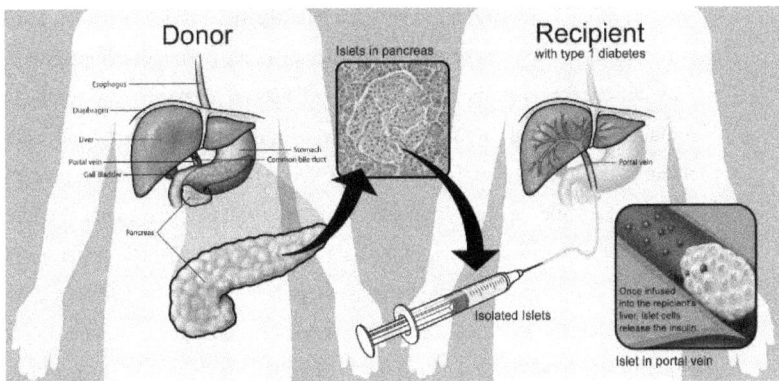

The primary thought of islet transplantation is to process the organ benefactors' pancreas to evacuate 95% of the organ liable for its exocrine capacities (discharge of stomach related proteins) and disengage the 5% of the organ answerable for the endocrine hormone emission the alleged pancreatic islets. When separated, the restorative group can imbue the insulin-creating islets through a flimsy cylinder, put in the primary vein that transports blood from the digestive organs to the liver. Once injected, the islets are shipped by the circulatory system into the liver, where they stop, take up living arrangement, and start making the perfect measure of insulin to control the glucose.

Current Limitations of Islet Transplantation

While huge advancement has been made in the islet transplantation field numerous deterrents remain that right now block its broad application. Two of the most significant restrictions are the as of now insufficient methods for forestalling islet dismissal, and the constrained stock of islets for transplantation. Current invulnerable suppressive regimens are fit for forestalling islet disappointment for quite a long time to years, yet the operators utilized in these medications are costly and may build the hazard for explicit malignancies and astute diseases. Likewise, and fairly unexpectedly, the most generally utilized specialists (like steroids, calcineurin inhibitors, and rapamycin) are likewise known to impede ordinary islet work and additionally insulin activity. Further, similar to all drugs, the specialists have other related toxicities, with symptoms, for example, oral ulcers, fringe edema, paleness, weight reduction, hypertension, hyperlipidemia, the runs, and exhaustion. Maybe of most noteworthy worry to the patient and doctor is the destructive impact of certain broadly utilized insusceptible suppressive specialists on renal capacity. For the patient with diabetes, renal capacity is a pivotal factor in deciding the long haul result, and calcineurin inhibitors (tacrolimus and cyclosporin) are fundamentally nephrotoxic. Accordingly, while a few patients with a pancreas transplant endure the immunosuppressive specialists well, and for such patients, diabetic nephropathy can continuously improve, in different patients, the net impact (diminished hazard because of the improved blood glucose control, expanded hazard from the immunosuppressive operators) may exacerbate kidney work. Surely, Ojo et al. have distributed an examination showing that among patients accepting other-than-kidney allografts, 7%–21% end up with renal disappointment because of the transplant or potentially Resulting immunosuppression.

Is Islet Transplantation Ready for Widespread Uses

While nobody recommends that the treatment is prepared for far reaching clinical application, another method for featuring current issues is to concentrate on cost. Expecting the present obstacles were cleared, islet transplantation costs around $150,000 per quiet per transplant. With more than 1 million Americans managing T1DM, it would cost over $100 billion to give every patient a solitary islet transplant, with little confirmation so far of any long haul advantage. Interestingly, the yearly immediate expense of a demonstrated treatment like concentrated insulin treatment is about $3,500 per persistent.

The long haul security and viability of the methodology stay vague.

The constraints of islet transplantation drive us to perceive that the treatment stays test and that numerous inquiries must be replied before it is consolidated into general clinical practice. At present, we encourage an emphasis on the choice of just those patients for whom this system offers the best probability of advantage. The vast majority with diabetes can, with determination and persistence, actualize an insulin routine that keeps up tight glucose control while staying away from risky hypoglycemia. In any case, a few patients keep on having gigantic trouble dealing with their ailment regardless of ideal consideration and exertion. Indeed, even the announcement "regardless of ideal consideration and exertion" is hard to characterize, and we advocate that all patients being considered for an islet transplant initially be alluded for a while to claim to fame groups that are focused on diabetes care. Since such patients whose diabetes is the most hard to control have a low quality of life, islet transplantation offers potential advantages. Indeed, even a low pattern level of insulin creation by the transplanted islets may bring down the measure of insulin required while diminishing the number and seriousness of hypoglycemic occasions. We likewise accept the islet transplant hazard advantage proportion is ideal for those with both T1DM and kidney disappointment who are recorded for a real existence safeguarding kidney transplant; such patients should take immunosuppressive operators after transplant to protect the kidney allograft work, so the islets can be included without an excessive amount of extra chance.

Similarly as early investigations indicated islet transplantation's guarantee, inquire about must presently beat the obstacles uncovered by the ongoing islet transplant understanding. New invulnerable modulatory specialists offer the best any desire for changing the field. New medication regimens equipped for prompting resilience to the transplanted islets would permit beneficiaries to keep up their unions without general invulnerable concealment and its related toxicities. While numerous objectives are as of now under scrutiny, none are prepared for clinical use. We advocate that such Immune modulatory approaches be tried first in quite a while where the outcomes can be suitably credited to the operator itself. Not exactly a century back, T1DM was a constantly deadly malady. With the approach of insulin, the guess changed medium-term, and we have kept on seeing upgrades in diabetes care and results. Pancreatic.

5. GENETICS OF DIABETES

Type 1 and type 2 diabetes contain different causes. Two variables are basic in both. Characteristics, yet nature also anticipate a basic action.

Qualities alone are insufficient. One proof of this is indistinguishable twins. Indistinguishable twins have indistinguishable qualities. However when one twin has type 1 diabetes, different gets the infection at most just a fraction of the time. At the point when one twin has type 2 diabetes, the other's hazard is all things considered 3 of every 4.

Type 1 Diabetes:

Much of the time, individuals need to acquire hazard factors from the two guardians. The vast majority who are in danger don't get diabetes and scientists need to discover what the natural triggers are.

Triggers:

- ✓ **Cold climate** - Type 1 diabetes grows more regularly in winter than summer and is increasingly normal in places with cold atmospheres (this condition is found in white individuals).

- ✓ **Viruses** - Perhaps an infection that has just gentle impacts on the vast majority triggers type 1 diabetes in others.

- ✓ **Early diet** - Type 1 diabetes is less basic in individuals who were breastfed and in the individuals who previously ate strong nourishments at later ages.

Scientists found that the vast majority of the individuals who later got diabetes had certain autoantibodies (antibodies that 'turned sour' which assault the body's tissues) in their blood for quite a long time previously.

Your Child's Risk:

PARENTS	RISK OF CHILD DEVELOPING DIABETES
Man with type 1 diabetes	1 in 17
Woman with type 1 diabetes (age below 25)	1 in 25
Woman with type 1 diabetes (age above 25)	1 in 100
A parent having Type 2 polyglandular autoimmune syndrome	1 in 2

Type 2 Polyglandular autoimmune syndrome - About 1 in every 7 people with type 1 diabetes has this condition. Notwithstanding having diabetes, these individuals likewise have thyroid malady and an ineffectively working adrenal organ. Some likewise have other invulnerable framework issue.

One of the most expensive tests that can be done for children who have siblings with type 1 diabetes. This test estimates antibodies to insulin, to islet cells in the pancreas, or to a compound called glutamic corrosive decarboxylase. Significant levels can show that a youngster has a higher danger of creating type 1 diabetes.

Type 2 Diabetes:

Type 2 diabetes has a more grounded connection to family ancestry and heredity than type 1, in spite of the fact that it also relies upon natural components. Studies of twins have shown that genetics plays a very strong role in the development of type 2 diabetes.

It may be very difficult to figure out whether diabetes is due to lifestyle factors or genetic susceptibility. Most likely it is due to both.

It is possible to delay or prevent type 2 diabetes by doing exercise and losing weight.

Risk factors for diabetes and progression to T2DM.

Risk factors for diabetes and progression to T2DM

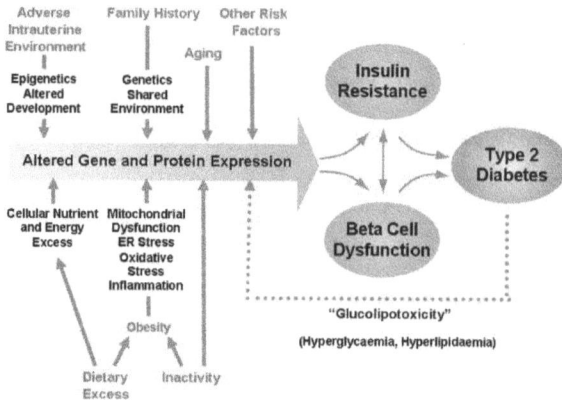

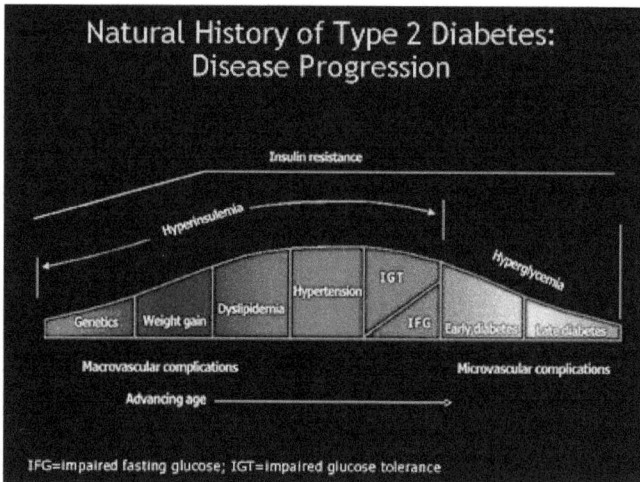

PARENTS	RISK OF CHILD DEVELOPING DIABETES
Man with type 2 diabetes (if diagnosed before age 50)	1 in 7
Man with type 2 diabetes (if diagnosed after age 50)	1 in 13
Mother with type 2 diabetes	Greater risk
Both parents with type 2 diabetes	1 in 2
MODY	1 in 2

*MODY - Maturity-Onset Diabetes of the Young. It is one of the uncommon sorts.

6. SIGNS AND SYMPTOMS OF DIABETES

NORMAL SIGNS AND SYMPTOMS OF DIABETES:

The most well-known signs and side effects of diabetes are

- ✓ Frequent pee
- ✓ Disproportionate thirst
- ✓ Intense hunger
- ✓ Weight gain
- ✓ Unusual weight reduction
- ✓ Increased weakness
- ✓ Irritability
- ✓ Blurred vision
- ✓ Cuts and wounds don't recuperate appropriately or rapidly
- ✓ More skin and additionally yeast contaminations
- ✓ Itchy skin
- ✓ Gums are red and additionally swollen
- ✓ Frequent gum illness/contamination

✓ Sexual brokenness (men)

✓ Numbness or shivering, particularly in your feet and hands

✓ We will analyze every one of these side effects in more detail underneath.

Frequent pee

When there is an excessive amount of glucose (sugar) in your blood you will see all the more regularly. On the off chance that your insulin is ineffectual, or not there by any means, your kidneys can't channel the glucose once again into the blood. The kidneys will take water from your blood to weaken the glucose - which thus tops off your bladder.

Lopsided thirst

On the off chance that you are peeing more than expected, you should supplant that lost fluid. You will drink more than expected.

Extreme yearning

As the insulin in your blood isn't working appropriately or isn't there in any way, and your cells are not getting their vitality, your body may respond by attempting to discover more vitality - nourishment. You will get ravenous.

Weight gain

This may be the aftereffect of the above manifestation (extreme yearning).

Uncommon weight reduction

This is progressively basic among individuals with Diabetes Type 1. As your body isn't making insulin it will search out another vitality source (the cells aren't getting glucose). Muscle tissue and fat will be separated for vitality. As Type 1 is of progressively abrupt beginning and Type 2 is substantially more continuous, weight reduction is increasingly perceptible with Type 1.

Expanded weakness

On the off chance that your insulin isn't working appropriately or isn't there in any way, glucose won't enter your cells and furnishing them with vitality. This will cause you to feel worn out and sluggish.

Crabbiness

Crabbiness can be because of your absence of vitality.

Obscured vision

This can be brought about by tissue being pulled from your eye focal points. This influences your eye's capacity to center. With legitimate treatment, this can be dealt with. There are serious situations where visual impairment or delayed vision issues can happen.

Cuts and wounds don't mend appropriately or rapidly. When there is more sugar (glucose) in your body, its capacity to mend can be undermined.

More skin or potentially yeast contaminations

When there is more sugar in your body, its capacity to recuperate from contaminations is influenced. Ladies with diabetes discover it particularly hard to recuperate from bladder and vaginal contaminations.

Irritated skin

A sentiment of irritation on your skin is here and there a manifestation of diabetes.

Gums are red and additionally swollen - gums pull away from teeth

On the off chance that your gums are delicate, red and additionally swollen this could be an indication of diabetes. Your teeth could turn out to be free as the gums pull away from them.

Visit gum ailment/disease

Just as the past gum indications, you may encounter increasingly visit gum malady as well as gum contaminations.

Sexual brokenness among men

On the off chance that you are more than 50 and experience continuous or steady sexual brokenness (erectile brokenness), it could be a side effect of diabetes.

Deadness or shivering, particularly in your feet and hands

In the event that there is an excessive amount of sugar in your body your nerves could get harmed, as could the little veins that feed those nerves. You may encounter shivering and additionally deadness in your grasp and feet.

Diabetic Coma

Trance state is generally uncommon in analyzed diabetes however it is critical to know about the circumstances that expansion the danger of trance like state. The primary driver of unconsciousness happening in individuals with diabetes are a consequence of extremely low or exceptionally high blood glucose levels.

There are three most basic reasons for trance like state in diabetic individuals:

✓ Severe hypoglycemia
✓ Diabetic ketoacidosis
✓ Hyperglycaemic hyperosmolar state

Diabetic trance states happen when an individual doesn't find a way to direct or adjust the glucose level when it is excessively high or excessively low. Glucose levels drop when the individual doesn't eat appropriately at once or when more insulin is taken. Glucose level may rise when a portion of insulin or different diabetes medicine is missed, when an eating regimen plan isn't followed appropriately, or when there is an absence of activity than expected. In individuals with diabetes blood, sugar may emerge during contaminations, hormone lopsided characteristics, and extreme diseases. High glucose for the most part makes advances on typical gradually than low glucose.

Diabetic extreme lethargies can happen because of a portion of the other not many variables like:

✓ When an insulin siphon doesn't work appropriately Injury, medical procedure, or another medical issue, for example, cardiovascular breakdown.

✓ When suppers are skipped or not insulin isn't taken.

✓ On taking liquor or unlawful medications.

Various, basically vascular intricacies may result because of Poorly controlled Hyperglycaemia. This influences little vessels (microvascular), enormous vessels (macrovascular), or both.

7. COMPLICATIONS OF DIABETES

Complications of Diabetes occur when

✓ Treatment isn't started

✓ The individual is experiencing type 1 diabetes

✓ Treatment isn't taken normally

✓ The tolerant isn't reacting to the treatment

✓ Dosage of medication or infusion is less or more than required

✓ Regular glucose or other screening tests are not done

✓ The ailment is available for a significant stretch particularly type 1

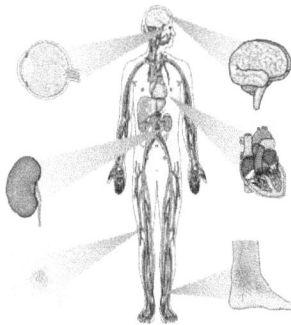

Major Complications of Diabetes

Microvascular

Eye
High blood glucose and high blood pressure can damage eye blood vessels, causing retinopathy, cataracts and glaucoma

Kidney
High blood pressure damages small blood vessels and excess blood glucose overworks the kidneys, resulting in nephropathy.

Neuropathy
Hyperglycemia damages nerves in the peripheral nervous system. This may result in pain and/or numbness. Feet wounds may go undetected, get infected and lead to gangrene.

Macrovascular

Brain
Increased risk of stroke and cerebrovascular disease, including transient ischemic attack, cognitive impairment, etc.

Heart
High blood pressure and insulin resistance increase risk of coronary heart disease

Extremities
Peripheral vascular disease results from narrowing of blood vessels increasing the risk for reduced or lack of blood flow in legs. Feet wounds are likely to heal slowly contributing to gangrene and other complications.

Complications linked to badly controlled diabetes:

The following is a rundown of potential complexities that can be brought about by gravely controlled diabetes:

- Eye inconveniences - glaucoma, waterfalls, diabetic retinopathy, and some others.

Normal   Glaucoma

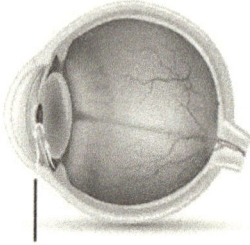

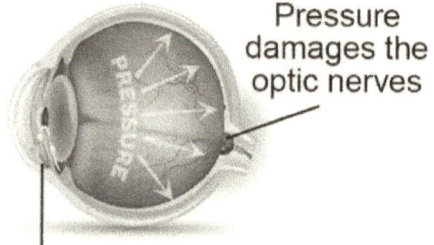

Pressure
damages the
optic nerves

Drainage canal allows
fluids to flow out

Drainage canal blocked,
fluid builds up in the eye

Glaucoma

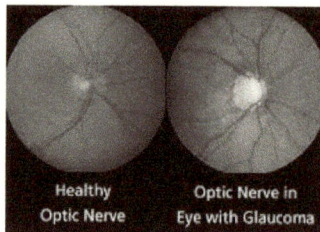

Healthy
Optic Nerve

Optic Nerve in
Eye with Glaucoma

Cataracts

Diabetic Retinopathy

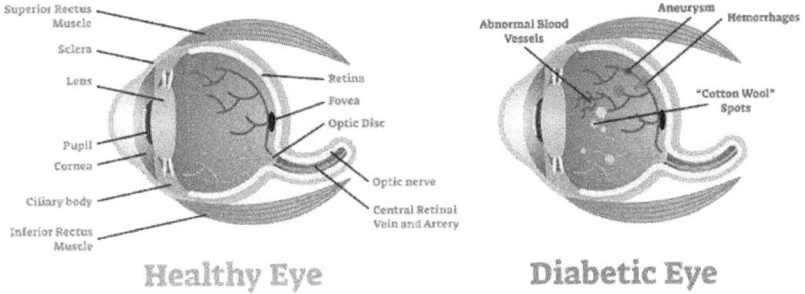

Healthy Eye   Diabetic Eye

DIABETIC RETINOPATHY

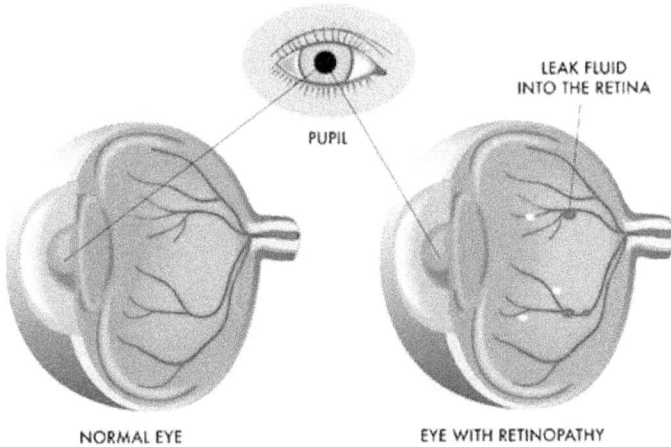

Diabetic retinopathy

- **Foot complications** - Neuropathy, ulcers, and now and then gangrene which may necessitate that the foot be removed.

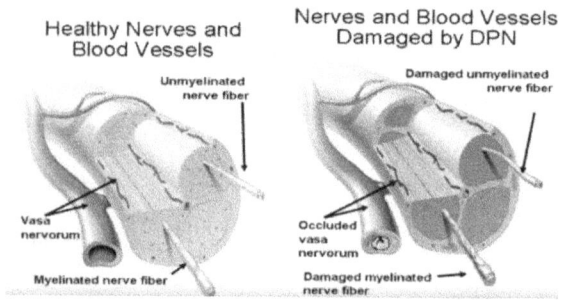

Healthy Nerves and Blood Vessels

Nerves and Blood Vessels Damaged by DPN

Unmyelinated nerve fiber

Damaged unmyelinated nerve fiber

Vasa nervorum

Occluded vasa nervorum

Myelinated nerve fiber

Damaged myelinated nerve fiber

- **Skin complications** - •individuals with diabetes are progressively vulnerable to skin diseases and skin issue

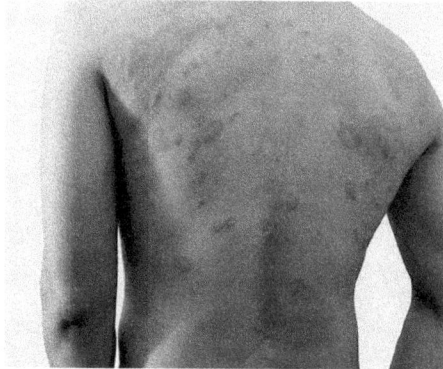

Skin rashes

• **Heart Problems -** For instance, ischemic coronary illness, when the blood supply to the guts muscle is reduced.

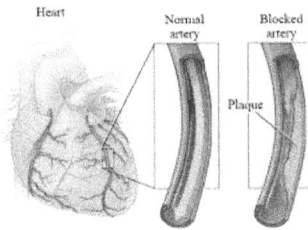

Ischemic heart disease

• **Hypertension** - normal in individuals with diabetes, which can bring up the danger of kidney malady, eye issues, cardiovascular failure and stroke.

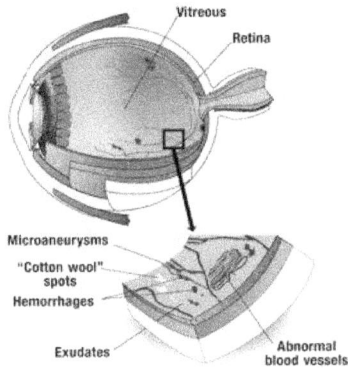

Hypertensive retinopathy

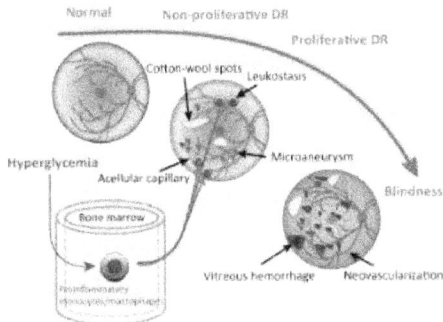

Heart attack

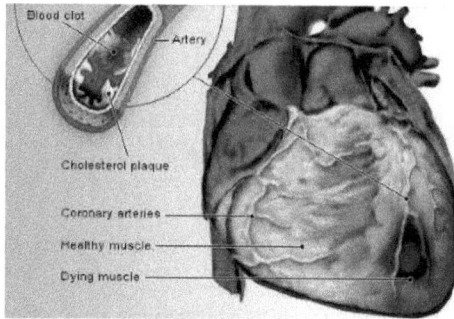

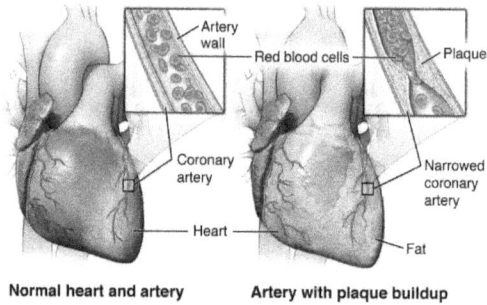

Normal heart and artery   **Artery with plaque buildup**

Stroke

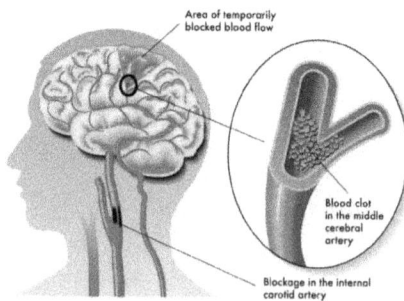

- **Mental wellbeing** - uncontrolled diabetes raises the danger of experiencing sorrow, tension and some other mental issue.

- **Hearing misfortune** - diabetes patients have a better danger of making hearing issues.

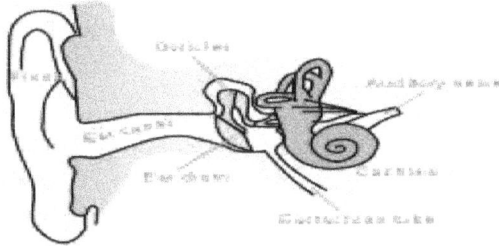

Hearing Loss

Gum ailment - there is an a lot higher commonness of gum illness among diabetes patients.

Periodontal ailment can prompt agonizing biting troubles and even tooth misfortune. Dry mouth, frequently a side effect of undetected diabetes, can cause irritation, ulcers, infections, and tooth rot. Smoking exacerbates these issues. Great blood glucose control is vital to controlling and forestalling mouth issues.

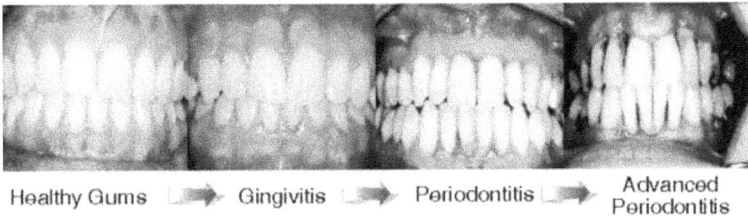

Healthy Gums ➡ Gingivitis ➡ Periodontitis ➡ Advanced Periodontitis

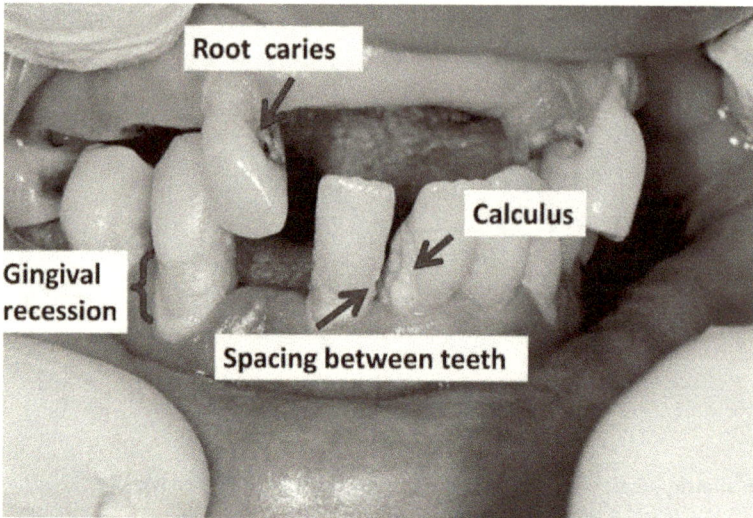

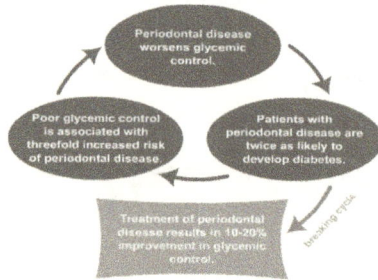

• **Gastroparesis** - the muscles of the stomach pack up properly.

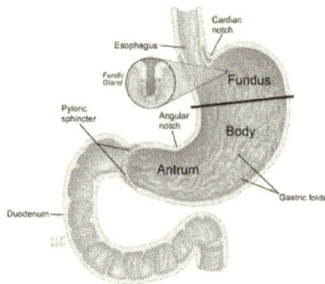

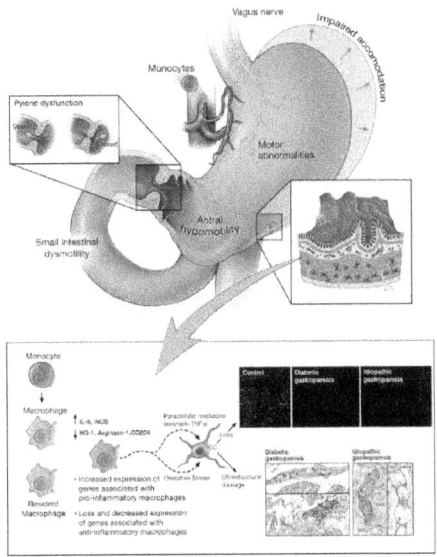

stomach pack

• **Ketoacidosis** - a mix of ketosis and acidosis; amassing of ketone bodies and corrosiveness in the blood.

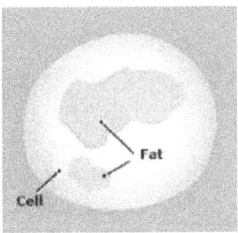

When glucose is used for fuel, the body stores fat for energy

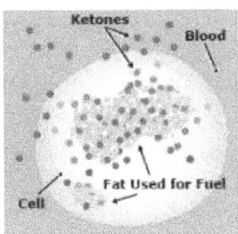

When fat is used for fuel, ketones are released into the blood

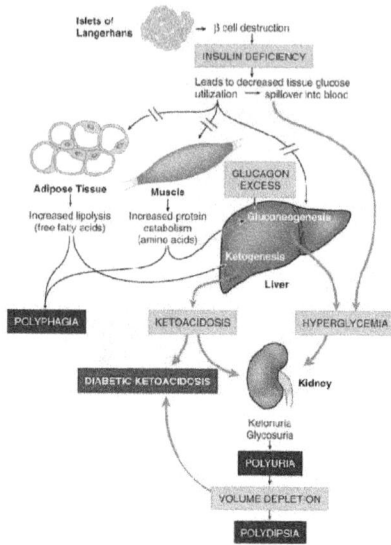

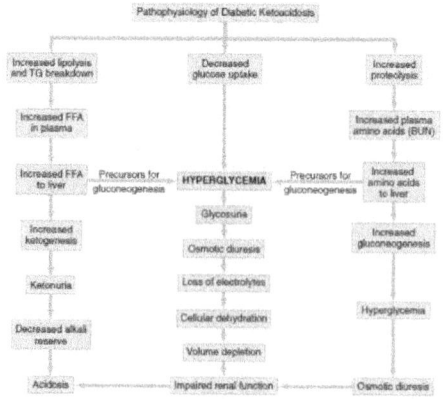

Pathophysiology map

FFA - Free Fatty Acids, TG - Triglycerides, BUN - Blood Urea Nitrogen

• **Neuropathy** - Diabetic neuropathy may be a kind of nerve harm which will prompt a couple of distinct issues.

Motor Neuropathy	• muscle weakness → foot drop • muscle imbalance → deformities
Sensory Neuropathy	• loss of feeling → loss of protective sensation, ulcers • loss of proprioception → poor balance
Autonomic Neuropathy	• loss of sweat (moisture) → dry cracked skin, ulcers • changes in blood flow → Charcot arthropathy

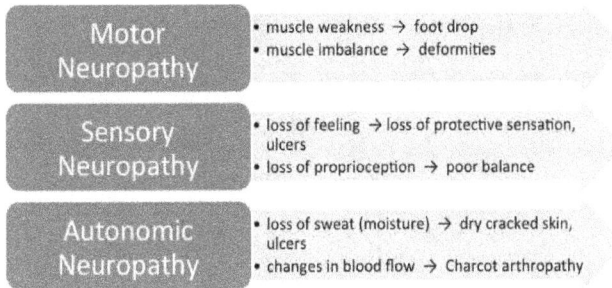

HHNS (Hyperosmolar Hyperglycemic Nonketotic Syndrome) - blood glucose levels shoot up unreasonably high, and there are no ketones present in the blood or pee. It is an emergency condition.

➢ **Nephropathy** - uncontrolled circulatory strain can prompt kidney illness.

➢ **PAD (fringe blood vessel malady)** - indications may remember torment for the leg, shivering and here and there issues strolling appropriately.

Claudication is torment brought about by too little blood stream to your legs or arms. This is typically a manifestation of fringe course illness.

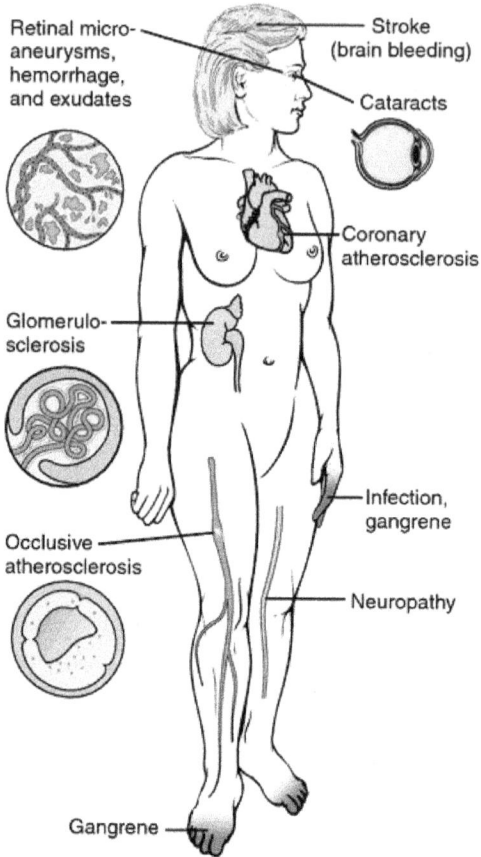

Retinal micro-
aneurysms,
hemorrhage,
and exudates

Stroke
(brain bleeding)

Cataracts

Coronary
atherosclerosis

Glomerulo-
sclerosis

Infection,
gangrene

Occlusive
atherosclerosis

Neuropathy

Gangrene

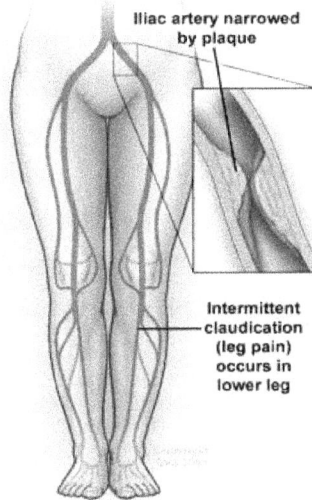

Iliac artery narrowed by plaque

Intermittent claudication (leg pain) occurs in lower leg

Claudication

➢ **Stroke** - Circulatory strain, cholesterol levels, and blood sugar levels aren't controlled, the danger of stroke increments fundamentally

➢ **Erectile brokenness** - male weakness. The nonappearance of erectness in the penis.

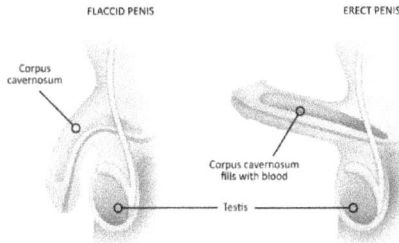

FLACCID PENIS

ERECT PENIS

Corpus cavernosum

Corpus cavernosum fills with blood

Testis

➢ **Infections** - individuals with gravely controlled diabetes are significantly more defenseless to diseases. The microscopic organisms, contagious and viral contaminations caused in diabetics and their treatment are clarified in detail and independently in the up and coming section.

> **Healing of wounds** - cuts and injuries take any longer to mend.

> **Thyroid issue** - Hyperthyroidism or Hypothyroidism were seen in diabetics.

Thyroid disorder and Diabetes

Thyroid disease and diabetes are both autoimmune disorders and may co-exist. In such a condition, if the thyroid disorder is left untreated, it could lead to difficulty in controlling the blood glucose levels.

Hyperthyroidism and Diabetes

The patient experiences tremors in the body because of an undetected overactive thyroid.

The patient may confuse it with low sugar levels

Consequently, the patient increases sugar intake to balance his glucose level.

This leads to high sugar levels, which further complicates the issue.

Note: Check your glucose level before you increase your sugar intake.

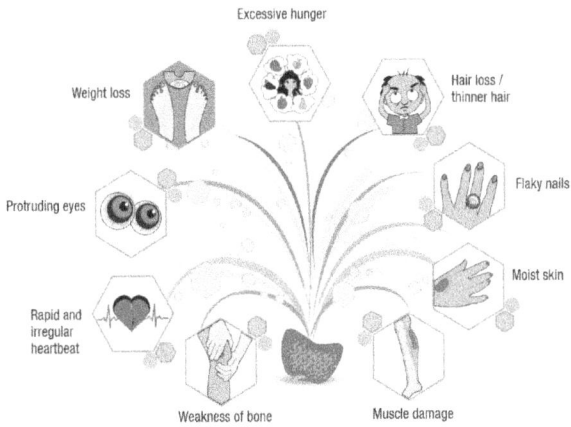

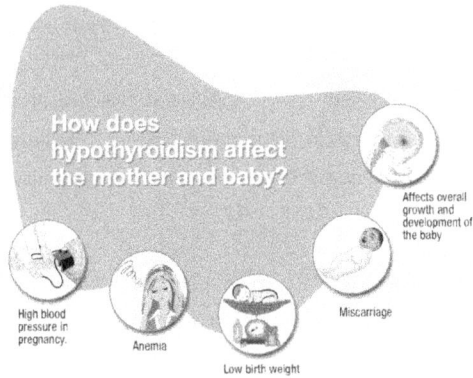

How does hypothyroidism affect the mother and baby?

High blood pressure in pregnancy.

Anemia

Low birth weight

Miscarriage

Affects overall growth and development of the baby

There are various therapeutic outcomes of industriously elevated levels of blood glucose. The most genuine include kidney disappointment, eye issues (visual impairment), neurological harm and expanded danger of cardiovascular issues (counting coronary failure and stroke).

A few side effects and cautioning signs are basic in both sort 1 and type 2 diabetes. These can be found in the table beneath and include: being exceptionally parched, visit pee, quick weight reduction, outrageous craving, shortcoming and weakness, ailment and peevishness.

8. TESTS AND DIAGNOSIS OF DIABETES

Criteria for Suspicion of Diabetes:

- ✓ In people matured 40 years or more.
- ✓ With a past filled with diabetes in a blood relative.
- ✓ Excessively overweight.
- ✓ Persons with side effects like expanded thirst, hunger and weight reduction, regardless of good nourishment admission, visit diseases, unexplained shortcoming.
- ✓ Persons with coronary illness, hypertension, unclear agonies in the body.
- ✓ Women who have gained over the top load during pregnancy.
- ✓ Women who have conveyed an infant gauging more than 3.5 Kg.
- ✓ Multiple passings of infants previously or after birth.

What is pre-diabetes?

Most by far of patients with type 2 diabetes at first had prediabetes. Their blood glucose levels were higher than typical, yet not sufficiently high to justify a diabetes finding. The cells in the body are getting impenetrable to insulin. This condition is additionally called marginal diabetes.

Studies have demonstrated that even at the prediabetes arrange, some harm to the circulatory framework and the heart may as of now have happened.

The most effective method to decide if you have diabetes, prediabetes or not one or the other specialists can decide if a patient has a typical digestion, prediabetes or diabetes in one of the accompanying various ways. The potential tests are

- ✓ The A1C test
- ✓ Glucose test
- ✓ FPG (fasting plasma glucose) test
- ✓ OGTT (oral glucose resilience test)
- ✓ Postprandial glucose test
- ✓ Random glucose test

A1C TEST:

What is the A1C test?

The A1C test is a blood test that gives data about an individual's normal degrees of blood glucose, additionally called glucose, in the course of recent months. The A1C test is some of the time called the hemoglobin A1c, HbA1c, or glycohaemoglobin test. The A1C test is the essential test utilized for diabetes the board and diabetes examine.

How does the A1C test work?

The A1C test depends on the connection of glucose to hemoglobin, the protein in red platelets that conveys oxygen. In the body, red platelets are continually shaping and biting the dust, yet commonly they live for around 3 months. Along these lines, the A1C test mirrors the normal of an individual's blood glucose levels in the course of recent months. The A1C test result is represented as a rate. The higher the rate, the higher an individual's blood glucose levels have been. A typical A1C level is beneath 5.7 percent.

✓ At any rate 6.5% methods diabetes
✓ Somewhere in the range of 5.7% and 5.99% methods prediabetes
✓ Under 5.7% methods typical

GLUCOSE TEST:

A glucose test is a kind of blood test used to choose the proportion of glucose in the blood. It is chiefly utilized in screening for prediabetes or diabetes. Patients are told not to expend anything other than water during the fasting time frame. Caffeine will likewise mutilate the outcomes. On the off chance that the individual eats during the period wherein the individual should have been fasting then they may show glucose levels that may make their PCP think the individual has or is at extended peril of having diabetes. In individuals previously having diabetes, blood glucose checking is utilized with visit interims in the administration of the condition.

There are a couple of various sorts of glucose tests:

(1) Fasting glucose (FBS), fasting plasma glucose (FPG):

- ✓ 8 or 12 or 14 hours within the wake of eating
- ✓ At least 126 mg/dl implies diabetes
- ✓ Between 100 mg/dl and 125.99 mg/dl implies prediabetes
- ✓ Less than 100 mg/dl implies ordinary
- ✓ A strange perusing following the FPG implies the patient has weakened fasting glucose (IFG)

(2) Glucose Tolerance Test: Continuous testing

- ✓ At least 200 mg/dl implies diabetes
- ✓ Between 140 and 199.9 mg/dl implies prediabetes
- ✓ Less than 140 mg/dl implies typical
- ✓ A strange perusing following the OGTT implies the patient has debilitated glucose resilience (IGT)

(3) Postprandial glucose test (PC): 2 hours in the wake of eating

A degree of < 7.8 mmol/l (140 mg/dl) an hour and a half after a feast is typical.

(4) Random glucose test

It is a glucose test taken from a non-fasting subject. This test, additionally called arbitrary blood glucose (RBG) or easygoing blood glucose (CBG) or irregular plasma glucose (RPG), accept an ongoing dinner and in this manner has higher reference esteems than the fasting glucose test.

Reference esteems

The reference esteems for a "typical" arbitrary glucose test in a normal grown-up are 79 - 140 mg/dl (4.4 - 7.8 mmol/l), between 140 - 200 mg/dl is considered pre-diabetes, and > 200 mg/dl is viewed as diabetes as indicated by ADA rules (you should visit your primary care physician or a facility for extra tests anyway as an irregular glucose of > 200 mg/dl doesn't really mean you are diabetic).

Blood test levels for the determination of diabetes and pre-diabetes are sketched out underneath.

Blood Test Levels For Diagnosis Of	A1C Test (Percent)	Fasting Plasma Glucose Test (mg/dL)	Oral Glucose Tolerance Test (mg/dL)
Diabetes	6.5 or above	126 or above	200 or above
Prediabetes	5.7 to 6.4	100 to 125	140 to 199
Normal	About 5	99 or below	139 or below

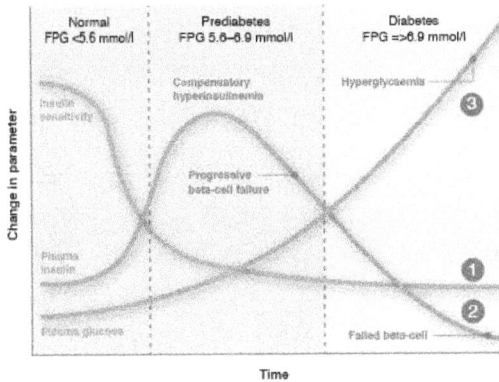

Recommended target blood sugar level ranges for non-diabetic and diabetes type 1 and type 2

For most of solid people, the ordinary blood glucose level in people is around 4 mmol/L or 72 mg/dL.

Target glucose levels by type	Glucose levels before meals	Glucose levels 2 hours after meals
Non-diabetic	4.0 to 5.9 mmol/L	Under 7.8 mmol/L
Diabetes type 2	4 to 7 mmol/L	Under 8.5 mmol/L
Diabetes type 1	4 to 7 mmol/L	Under 9 mmol/L
Children with diabetes type 1	4 to 8 mmol/L	Under 10 mmol/L

Pee EXAMINATION:

Pee is analyzed for the location of glucose (sugar) and ketones. Numerous tests are utilized for this reason.

(1) BENEDICT'S TEST:

This is the most established test used to identify diabetes. It is utilized uniquely in remote essential wellbeing habitats, where offices for different tests are not accessible. In a test tube, 8 drops of pee are blended in with 5 ml of Benedict's Qualitative arrangement, bubbled and shading noted.

The shade of the mix fills in as a manual for the proportion of sugar in the pee: blue-sugar missing; clear green - 0.1% sugar; turbid green - 0.3% sugar; green-0.5% sugar; yellow-1% sugar; orange-1.5% sugar; square red-2 % or more sugar.

The above test must be performed 2 hours after a feast. In the underlying phases of the sickness, a diabetic doesn't lose sugar in his pee, when on void stomach. Henceforth if Benedict's test is acted in the fasting state, it is conceivable to miss the finding of the infection. Regardless of whether sugar is distinguished in the pee by Benedict's test, the conclusion of diabetes ought to be affirmed by blood examination.

Detriments:

- ✓ It gives just an unrefined thought of diabetes, since it uncovers the nearness of sugar, just when glucose expands in excess of 180 mg %. for example in instances of extreme diabetes.
- ✓ Even if different sugars, for example fructose, galactose, maltose and lactose are found in pee, the test gives positive outcomes.
- ✓ Certain drugs like ibuprofen, penicillin, different anti-infection agents and Vitamin C can likewise give positive outcomes.
- ✓ In kids, gathering a pee test is troublesome.

(2) DIPSTICK TEST:

A pee test strip or dipstick test is a fundamental symptomatic apparatus used to decide neurotic changes in a patient's pee in standard urinalysis. There are sure paper or plastic strips covered with synthetics that change hues as indicated by sugar and ketone focuses. For instance, one kind of strip ranges from yellow through green to dim blue and another from blue through green to dark colored. The dipstick is dunked in new pee or straightforwardly through the pee stream and inside 30 seconds, the shading change is contrasted and the shading diagram given on the compartment.

Preferences:

✓ Very straightforward method.
✓ The result is immediate.
✓ User-accommodating and the patient at home can do it effectively.

Detriments:

✓ The strips are expensive.
✓ Patients with partial blindness may confuse the outcomes.
✓ Vitamin C and different prescriptions may meddle with the outcomes.

Identification OF KETONES:

(2) ROTHERA'S TEST:

It is otherwise called Rothera nitroprusside test. 5 mL of crisp pee is soaked with strong ammonium sulfate and blended in with 10 drops of newly arranged 2% sodium nitroprusside arrangement. At that point 10 drops of concentrated smelling salts water are included through the sides of the test cylinder and permitted to represent 15 minutes; the nearness of acetoacetic corrosive, or bigger groupings of CH3)2CO, is shown by the advancement of a blue-purple shading ring at the intersection.

(3) GERHARDT'S TEST:

5 ml of the crisp pee test is taken in a perfect test tube and a 10% FeCl3 arrangement is included dropwise and watched for the development of any red-dark colored encourage.

Examination of tests and determination for diabetes type 1 and diabetes type 2

	Diabetes type 1	Diabetes type 2
Conceivable reason factors	• Genetic • Environmental • Autoimmune factors • Idiopathic.	• Genetic • Obesity • Physical latency • High/low birth weight • Gestational diabetes mellitus (GDM) • Poor placental development Metabolic • Metabolic disorder.
Normally distressed gatherings (yet not elite to)	• Children Teens.	• Adults • Elderly • Certain ethnic gatherings.
Inclined ethnic groups	• All.	• African-American • Latino/Hispanic • Native American • Asian • Pacific Islander.
Prevalence	• 5%	• 95%
Influenced age group	• Typically age 5 - 25 (can influence individuals of any age).	• Most normal in grown-ups, yet can likewise create around adolescence. Most kids with type 2 diabetes have a family ancestry of diabetes, are overweight, and are not truly dynamic. As of not long ago, just sort 1 diabetes was regularly analyzed in youngsters
Test	• A1C test • Random plasma glucose • Fasting plasma glucose • Genetic testing is	• A1C test • Random plasma glucose • Fasting plasma glucose • Oral glucose resistance tests may likewise be led (infrequently).

	led in situations where there is a family ancestry of the disease.	

These days, huge numbers of the medical clinics are giving expert wellbeing exams to diabetic patients. These tests can be taken by the patient at any rate once per year. They are as per the following:

(1) DIABETIC PROFILE:

The diabetic profile test incorporates Fasting Serum Glucose, Post Prandial Plasma Glucose and Glycosylated Hemoglobin (HbA1c). There are various techniques to play out these tests. One of the models is given underneath with the standard reference esteems for diabetics.

Tests	Reference range
Fasting Serum Glucose (Hexokinase method)	70 to 100 mg/dl (3.9 to 5.6 mmol/l)
Post-Prandial Plasma Glucose (Hexokinase method)	120 to 140 mg/dl (6.7 to 7.8 mmol/l)
Glycosylated Haemoglobin (HbA1c) by HPLC (High-Performance Liquid Chromatography) method	less than 7.0 %

(2) LIPID PROFILE:

Coming up next are the reference esteems given by the acclaimed Diabetes Research Institute and Diabetes Care Center at Chennai.

Tests	Reference range
Total Cholesterol (GPO-PAP)	<=200 mg/dl
HDL Cholesterol (High-Density Lipoprotein) - Direct	>=40 mg/dl
LDL Cholesterol (Low-Density Lipoprotein) - Calculated	<=100 mg/dl
VLDL Cholesterol - Calculated	Up to 30 mg/dl

Triglycerides (GPO-PAP)	<=150 mg/dl
The ratio of CHOL / HDL	<4.5

(3) RENAL PROFILE:

Tests	Reference range
Urea (Urease/Glutamate dehydrogenase method)	15 to 45 mg/dl
Creatinine (Jaffe Rate Blanked method)	0.6 to 1.2 g/dl
Microalbumin/Creatinine ratio	Normal - <30 mg/alb/g
	Microalbuminuria - 30 to 229
	Macroalbuminuria - >300

Microalbuminuria is characterized as discharge of 30–300 mg of egg whites per 24 hours (or 20–200 mcg/min or 30–300 mcg/mg creatinine) on 2 of 3 pee assortments. The location of low degrees of egg whites discharge (microalbuminuria) has been connected to the ID of nascent diabetic kidney infection. This stage calls for forceful administration to forestall or impede clear diabetic nephropathy.

(4) RENAL FUNCTION TEST:

Tests	Reference range
Uric Acid (Uricase method)	Male - 2.5 to 7 mg/dl
	Female - 1.5 to 6 mg/dl

(5) LIVER FUNCTION TEST (LFT):

Tests	Reference range
Serum Bilirubin-Total (Diazotization method)	0.1 to 0.2 mg/dl
Serum Bilirubin-Direct (Diazotization method)	up to 0.2 mg/dl
Alkaline Phosphatase (IFCC method)	20 to 130 IU/L
SGOT (Serum Glutamic Oxaloacetic Transaminase) also called as AST (Aspartate	Male - <35 IU/L
	Female - <31 IU/L

Aminotransferase) by IFCC method without PP	
SGPT (Serum Glutamic Pyruvate Transaminase) also called as ALT (Alanine Transaminase) by IFCC method without PP	*Male - <45 IU/L* *Female - <34 IU/L*
GGTP (Gamma Glutamyl Transpeptidase) by Liquid stand IFCC method	*Male - <55 IU/L* *Female - <38 IU/L*
Total Proteins (Biuret method)	*6 to 8.5 g/dl*

Note:

1. SGOT - Normal serum contains just a limited quantity of GOT. It is available in bounty in heart muscles. It is additionally found in skeletal muscles. This level increments in states of broad harms to muscles particularly cardiovascular muscles. The estimation of SGOT is to affirm the determination of myocardial dead tissue.

2. SGPT - Normal serum contains just a limited quantity of GPT. Liver tissue is rich in GPT. SGPT level increments in patients with intense hepatic sickness, where liver cells are harmed. SGPT is viewed as an increasingly explicit record of hepatocellular harm.

3. GGTP (Gamma Glutamyl Transpeptidase) otherwise called GGT, assists with distinguishing liver and bile conduit damage just as incessant liquor misuse. In the event that GGT is ordinary in an individual with a high ALP, the reason is an in all probability bone sickness. GGT is an expansion in many infections that cause intense harm to the liver or bile channels.

(6) HAEMOGRAM COMPLETE:

Tests	*Reference range*
Hemoglobin	*Male - 13.5 to 17.5 g/dL* *Female - 11.5 to 16.5 /dL*

RBC Count	*Male - 4.7 to 6.1 million cells for every microliter (cells/mcL)* *Female - 4.2 to 5.4 million cells for each microliter (cells/mcL)*
Haematocrit	*Male - 40 to 52 %* *Female - 38 to 45 %*
MCV	*76 to 96 fl*
MCH	*27 to 31 pg*
MCHC	*32 to 36 gHb/100 ml*
Total WBC Count	*4,000 to 11,000 cells/mcL*
1. Neutrophils	*45 to 70 %*
2. Lymphocytes	*25 to 40 %*
3. Eosinophils	*1 to 6 %*
4. Monocytes	*2 to 8 %*
5. Basophils	*0 to 1 %*
PLATELET Count	*1,50,000 to 4,50,000 cells/mcL*

Note:

1. Haematocrit (Hct or PCV) - It is an estimation of the extent of blood that is comprised of cells. The worth is communicated as a small amount of cells in the blood. PCV is a Packed Cell Volume.

2. Mean Corpuscular Volume or Mean Cell Volume (MCV) - It is communicated in femtoliters (fl or 10-15 L)

$$MCV = \frac{\text{Hematocrit (\%) x 10}}{\text{RBC Count (millions/mm3 blood)}}$$

3. Mean Corpuscular Hemoglobin (MCH) - It is communicated in picograms per cell.

$$MCH = \frac{\text{Hb}}{\text{RBC}}$$

4. Mean Corpuscular Hemoglobin Concentration (MCHC) - It is communicated as grams of hemoglobin per 100 ml stuffed cells.

MCHC = $\dfrac{\text{Haemoglobin (g/100ml)} \times 100}{\text{Haematocrit (\%)}}$

Erythrocytes that have a typical size or volume (ordinary MCV) are called normocytic.

At the point when the MCV is high, it is called macrocytic.

At the point when the MCV is low, it is named microcytic.

Erythrocytes containing the ordinary measure of hemoglobin (typical MCHC) are called normochromic.

At the point when the MCHC is strangely low they are called hypochromic, and when the MCHC is unusually high, hyperchromic.

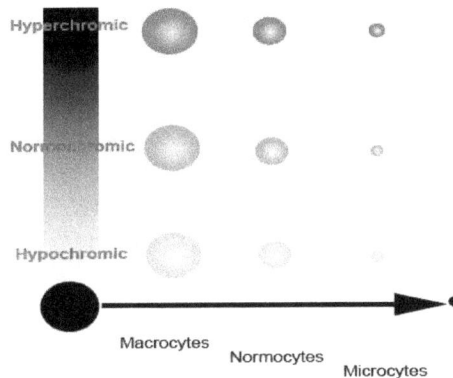

The terms above are utilized together to portray various types of iron deficiency. For instance, iron insufficiency frailty is depicted as microcytic and hypochromic, while nutrient B12 lack is macrocytic and normochromic.

(7) THYROID TEST:

Tests	Reference range
Thyroid Stimulating Hormone TSH (CLIA method - ChemiLuminescence ImmunoAssay)	*0.27 to 4.20 µIU/ml*

Thyroxine is the hormone emitted by the thyroid organ. It is put away in the colloid of the thyroid follicles, as a glycoprotein called thyroglobulin. Thyroxine assumes a significant job in starch, protein and lipid digestion. In starch digestion, thyroxine expands the pace of retention of monosaccharides by the digestive system; improves hepatic glycogenolysis, in this way expanding the glucose focus and furthermore favors gluconeogenesis. Every one of these variables add to the hyperglycemic condition of hyperthyroidism. The maladies related with irregular digestion of thyroxine are Hyperthyroidism and Hypothyroidism.

Thyroid Stimulating Hormone (TSH) is a thyrotropic hormone emitted by the foremost pituitary. It is a glycoprotein and has a high cysteine content. TSH assumes a significant job in the guideline of the emission of thyroxine. The emission of TSH by the front pituitary, then again, is constrained by the degree of coursing thyroxine. An expansion in the centralization of circling thyroxine discourages TSH creation. The abatement in the amount of flowing thyroxine expands TSH generation.

(8) VITAMIN D (TOTAL):

The 25-hydroxy nutrient D test is the most precise approach to gauge how a lot of nutrient D is in your body. In the kidney, 25-hydroxy nutrient D changes into a functioning type of the nutrient. The dynamic type of nutrient D helps control calcium and phosphate levels in the body. It is communicated as nanogram per milliliter.

	Nutrient D Council	Endocrine Society	Food and Nutrition Board	Testing Laboratories
Deficient	*0-30 ng/ml*	*0-20 ng/ml*	*0-11 ng/ml*	*0-31 ng/ml*
Insufficient	*31-39 ng/ml*	*21-29 ng/ml*	*12-20 ng/ml*	

Sufficient	40-80 ng/ml	30-100 ng/ml	>20 ng/ml	32-100 ng/ml
Toxic	>150 ng/ml			

(9) FOOT EXAMINATION:

✓ **Biothesiometry:**

The Bio-Thesiometer is an instrument planned to quantify fundamentally and very well the edge of energy about vibration in human subjects. It is a basic and practical device for the estimation of Vibration Perception Threshold.

The Bio-Thesiometer is used as an exploration gadget in numerous neurological sicknesses. More the VPT, more the danger of ulceration for a diabetic foot. This has manual control for applying vibration; it decreases the testing time by arriving at near the foreseen level quicker. One can then progressively increment or diminishing the voltages applied for the exact recognition of VPT. This likewise helps in keeping the instrument straightforward and financially savvy.

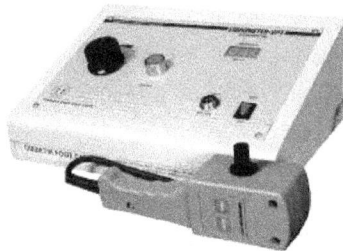

Bio-Thesiometer

✓ **Sensitometry**:

Sensitometer can cool to approach frosty temperatures and warming is limited to 49° Centigrade. It has different modes to test the limits. More straightforward modes help to immediately screen the patients. Complex calculations might be utilized as an amazing examination device. Thinking about the foot geometry and for a superior reaction for heat torment in the beginning periods ofneuropathy, a roundabout respectable metal test tip is utilized with hard gold plating.

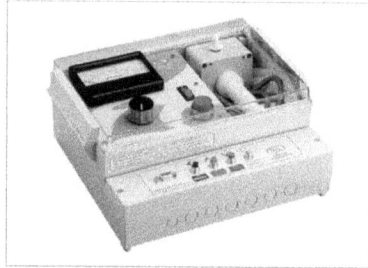

Sensitometer

✓ **Doppler Ultrasound Scan:**

A Doppler ultrasound is a test that utilizations high-recurrence sound waves (ultrasound) to gauge the measure of blood move through conduits and veins, for the most part those that supply blood to arms and legs. During the test, a water-dissolvable gel is put on a handheld gadget called a transducer. This gadget guides high-recurrence sound waves to the corridor or veins being tried. Circulatory strain sleeves might be put around various pieces of the body, including the thigh, calf, lower leg, and various focuses along the arm. A glue is applied to the skin over the supply routes being inspected. Pictures are made as the transducer is moved over every territory.

This test is to analyze arteriosclerosis (a narrowing and solidifying of the conduits that supply blood to the legs and feet), blood cluster called profound vein thrombosis (a condition that happens when a blood coagulation shapes in a vein somewhere inside body for the most part in the leg or hip locales), shallow thrombophlebitis (an aggravation of the veins because of a blood coagulation in a vein just underneath the skin's surface), thromboangiitis obliterans (an uncommon malady where the veins of the hands and feet become kindled and swollen) and vascular tumors in arms or legs.

Arteriosclerosis

An ordinary outcome implies the veins give no indications of narrowing, clusters, or conclusion, and the conduits have typical blood stream. Strange outcomes might be because of blockage in a supply route by a blood coagulation, blood cluster in a vein (DVT), narrowing or widening of a course, spastic blood vessel ailment (blood vessel constrictions expedited by cold or feeling), venous impediment (shutting of a vein), venous reflux (blood stream going the wrong bearing in veins) and blood vessel impediment from atherosclerosis.

Atherosclerosis

A few variables may bargain the outcomes, which implies the test will should be done once more. These components incorporate smoking short of what one hour before the test, serious corpulence, cardiovascular dysrhythmias and arrhythmias, or unpredictable heart rhythms and cardiovascular infection.

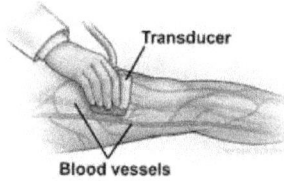

Transducer

Blood vessels

Foot Pressure Measurement System:

This framework rapidly catches static and dynamic estimations for foot work appraisals, curve portrayals, in-underside suggestions, top weights areas and surveying steadiness. Numerous privately owned businesses are giving these kinds of estimating frameworks. Model - Tekscan organization gives a foot pressure measuring system to diagnosing foot work in diabetics.

Low profile mat to capture barefoot pressures/forces

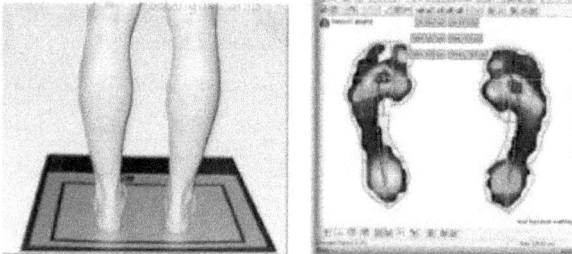

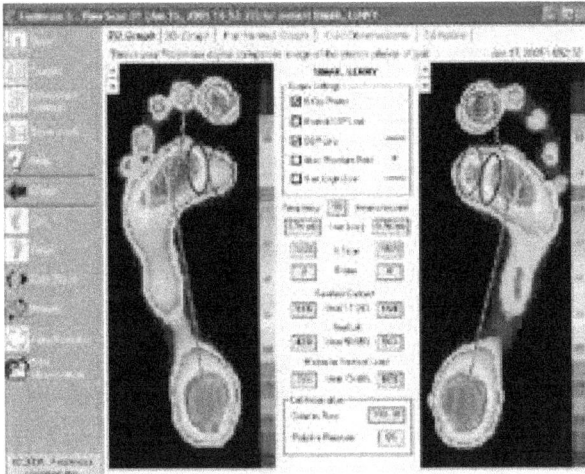

(10) ELECTROCARDIOGRAM (ECG or EKG):

The electrocardiogram (ECG or EKG) is a demonstrative apparatus that is routinely used to survey the electrical and solid elements of the heart. While it is a generally basic test to perform, the understanding of the ECG following requires noteworthy measures of preparing.

The heart is a two-arrange electrical siphon and the heart's electrical action can be measured by terminals set on the skin. The electrocardiogram can gauge the rate and mood of the heartbeat, just as give roundabout proof of blood stream to the heart muscle.

An institutionalized framework has been created for the cathode position for a standard ECG. Ten anodes are expected to create 12 electrical perspectives on the heart. Anelectrode lead, or fix, is set on each arm and leg and six are set over the chest divider. The signs got from every cathode are recorded. The printed perspective on these chronicles is the electrocardiogram.

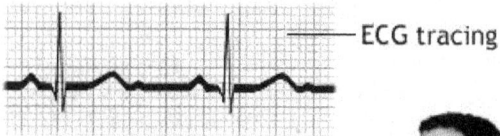

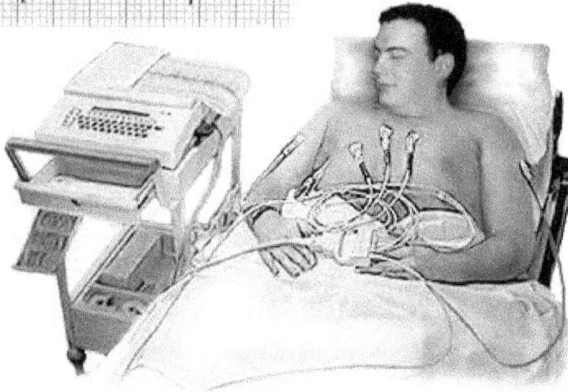

ECG tracing

Normal ECG

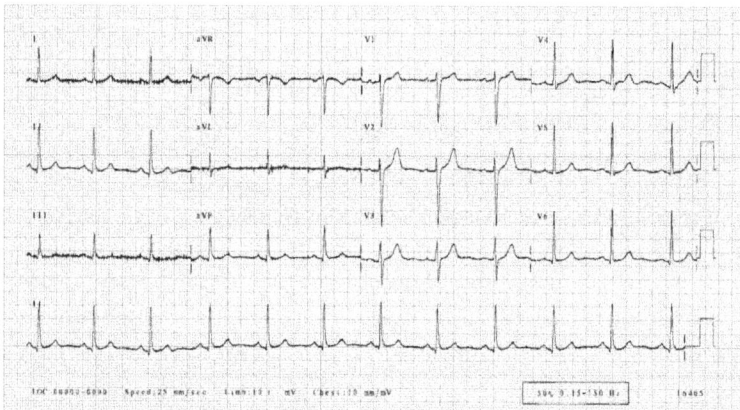

(11) ECHOCARDIOGRAPHY/ECHOCARDIOGRAM (ECHO):

An echocardiogram (reverberation) is a test that utilizations high-recurrence sound waves (ultrasound) to take photos of the heart. The test is additionally called echocardiography or analytic cardiovascular ultrasound. A reverberation utilizes sound waves to make photos of the heart's chambers, valves, dividers and the veins (aorta, supply routes, veins) appended to the heart.

70

A test called a transducer is mistreated your chest. The test produces sound waves that bob off your heart and "reverberation" back to the test. These waves are changed into pictures saw on a video screen. There are no unsafe reactions.

This test assists with discovering

✓ The size and state of your heart, and the size, thickness and development of your heart's dividers
✓ How your heart moves.
✓ The heart's siphoning quality.
✓ If the heart valves are working effectively.
✓ If blood is releasing in reverse through your heart valves (disgorging).
✓ If the heart valves are excessively thin (stenosis).
✓ If there is a tumor or irresistible development around your heart valves.
✓ Problems with the external coating of your heart (the pericardium).
✓ Problems with the huge veins that enter and leave the heart.
✓ Blood clumps in the assemblies of your heart.
✓ Abnormal gaps between the assemblies of the heart.

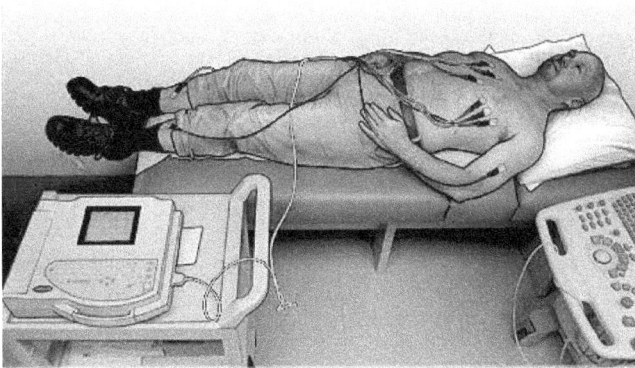

© Healthwise, Incorporated

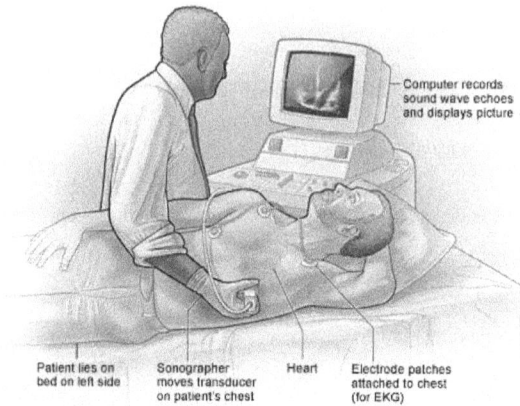

| Patient lies on bed on left side | Sonographer moves transducer on patient's chest | Heart | Electrode patches attached to chest (for EKG) |

Computer records sound wave echoes and displays picture

(12) TREADMILL EXERCISE STRESS TEST:

This test is additionally called a Cardiac Stress test. A treadmill practice pressure test is utilized to decide the impacts of activity on the heart. Exercise permits specialists to distinguish unusual heart rhythms (arrhythmias) and analyze the nearness or nonattendance of coronary supply route sickness. This test includes strolling set up on a treadmill while observing the electrical action of your heart. All through the test, the speed and slope of the treadmill increment. The outcomes show how well your heart reacts to the pressure of various degrees of activity. The method of this test as follows:

✓ You will be approached to expel all chest area dress, and to put on an outfit with the opening to the front.

✓ Adhesive anodes will be put onto your chest to catch an ECG. The destinations where the terminals are set will be cleaned with liquor and shaved if essential. A gentle scraped area may likewise be utilized to guarantee a decent quality ECG recording.

✓ Your resting circulatory strain, pulse, and ECG will be recorded.

✓ You will be approached to stroll on a treadmill. The walk begins gradually, at that point the speed and slope increments at set occasions. You should stroll to the extent that this would be possible on the grounds that the test is exertion subordinate.

✓ You will be checked all through the test. On the off chance that an issue happens, the technologist will stop the test immediately. You have to tell the technologist on the off chance that you experience any manifestations, for example, chest torment, wooziness, bizarre brevity of breath, or outrageous weariness.

72

✓ Following the test, you will be approached to rests. Your circulatory strain, pulse, and ECG will be observed for three to five minutes after exercise.

✓ The information will be looked into by a cardiologist after the test is finished. A report will be sent to the doctor(s) engaged with your consideration.

In the event that patients are utilizing Viagra, Cialis and Levitra, they are told to stop 48 hours before the test. Try not to eat, drink or smoke for 2 hours before the test. Take your standard meds except if in any case coordinated by your doctor. Carry the entirety of your meds with you in the first jugs. Wear agreeable garments and shoes that are appropriate for strolling on a treadmill. There are no limitations after the treadmill practice pressure test.

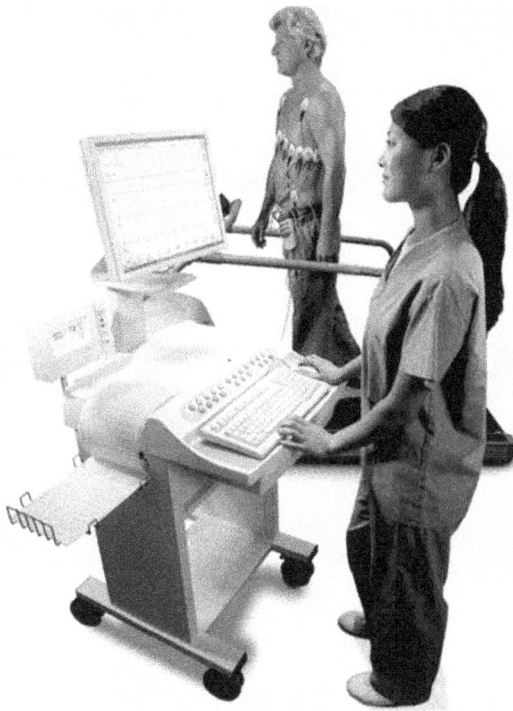

(13) X-RAY RADIOGRAPHY (CHEST):

A chest x-beam utilizes an extremely little portion of ionizing radiation to create photos of within the chest. It is utilized to assess the lungs, heart and chest divider and might be utilized to help analyze brevity of breath, persevering hack, fever, chest torment or damage. It additionally might be utilized to help analyze and screen treatment for an assortment of lung conditions, for example, pneumonia, emphysema and malignancy. Since chest x-beam is quick and simple, it is especially helpful in crisis finding and treatment.

Advantages:

✓ No radiation stays in a patient's body after a x-beam assessment.
✓ X-beams as a rule have no symptoms in the run of the mill symptomatic range for this test.
✓ X-beam gear is moderately reasonable and broadly accessible in crisis rooms, doctor workplaces, walking care focuses, nursing homes and different areas, making it advantageous for the two patients and doctors.
✓ Because x-beam imaging is quick and simple, it is especially helpful in crisis finding and treatment.

Dangers:

✓ There is constantly a slight possibility of disease from exorbitant presentation to radiation. In any case, the advantage of an exact finding far exceeds the hazard.
✓ The viable radiation portion for this system shifts.
✓ Women ought to consistently advise their doctor or x-beam technologist if there is any likelihood that they are pregnant.

Impediments:

The chest x-beam is a helpful assessment, yet it has confinements. Since certain states of the chest can't be distinguished on a customary chest x-beam picture, this assessment can't really preclude all issues in the chest. For instance, little tumors may not appear on a chest x-beam. A blood coagulation in the lungs, a condition called an aspiratory embolism, can't be seen on chest x-beams.

Further imaging examinations might be important to explain the consequences of a chest x-beam or to search for variations from the norm not unmistakable on the chest x-beam.

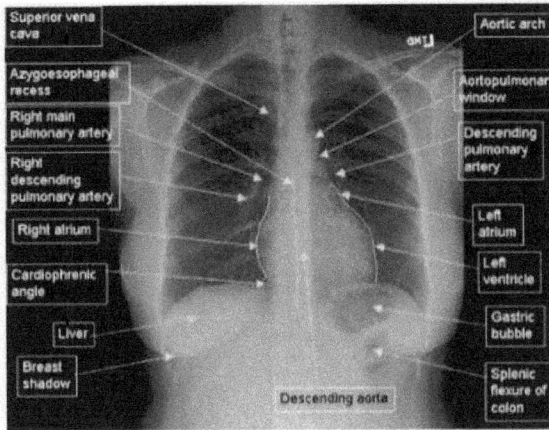

Normal X-Ray Chest

(14) ABDOMINAL ULTRASOUND:

A stomach ultrasound is a kind of imaging test. It is utilized to take a gander at organs in the belly, including the liver, gallbladder, spleen, pancreas, and kidneys. The veins that lead to a portion of these organs, for example, the second rate vena cava and aorta, can likewise be analyzed with ultrasound. A ultrasound machine makes pictures of organs and structures inside the body. The machine conveys high-recurrence sound waves that reflect off body structures. A PC gets these waves and uses them to make an image. Ultrasound is sheltered, noninvasive and doesn't utilize ionizing radiation. You will rests for the strategy.

A reasonable, water-based leading gel is applied to the skin over the stomach area. This assists with the transmission of the sound waves. A handheld test called a transducer is then moved over the guts. You may need to change position so the medicinal services supplier can take a gander at various regions. You may likewise need to hold your breath for brief periods during the test. More often than not, the test takes under 30 minutes.

This test is performed to

- ✓ Find the reason for stomach torment
- ✓ Find the reason for kidney contaminations
- ✓ Diagnose and screen tumors and malignant growths

- ✓ Diagnose or treat ascites (develop of liquid in the space between the covering of the mid-region and stomach organs)
- ✓ Learn why there is growing of a stomach organ
- ✓ Look for harm after damage
- ✓ Look for stones in the gallbladder or kidney
- ✓ Look for the reason for irregular blood tests, for example, liver capacity tests or kidney tests
- ✓ Look for the reason for a fever. The strange ultrasound can demonstrate conditions such
- ✓ Gallstones
- ✓ Kidney stones
- ✓ Pancreatitis (irritation in pancreas)
- ✓ Splenomegaly (Spleen broadening)
- ✓ Liver tumors
- ✓ Cirrhosis

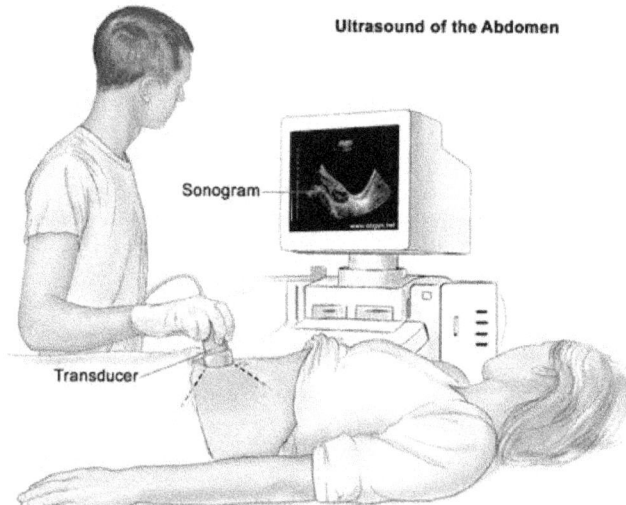

Ultrasound of the Abdomen

Sonogram

Transducer

Organ	Findings
Gallbladder, AB	Normal, thickening of wall, stones
Liver, AB	Normal, tumor, abscess, cysts
Pancreas, AB	Normal, inflammation, cysts
Abdominal aorta, AB	Normal, aneurysm
Kidneys, AB	Normal, hydronephrosis, cysts
Appendix, AB	Normal, thickening of wall (>3 mm), abscess
Colon diverticula, AB	Normal, thickening of wall (>3 mm), abscess
Bladder, AB/VG	Normal, urinary retention, stones, tumor
Ovaries, VG	Normal, cysts >25 mm
Uterus, VG	Normal, fibromas, thickening of the endometrium, intrauterine pregnancy
Small pelvis, VG	Normal, fluid in the Pouch of Douglas, tumor

AB - Abdominal Ultrasound

VG - Vaginal Ultrasound

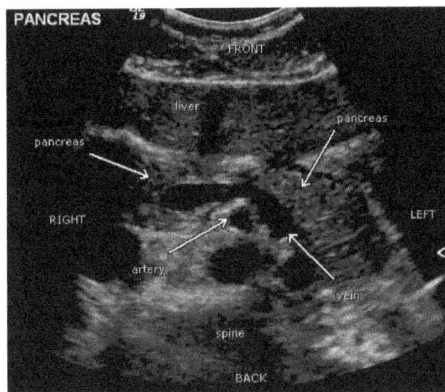

Ultrasound – Pancreas

Anatomy of the Human Eye

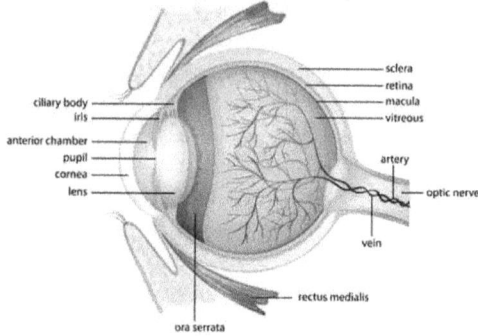

sclera
retina
macula
vitreous

ciliary body
iris

anterior chamber
pupil
cornea
lens

artery

optic nerve

vein

rectus medialis

ora serrata

Diabetic Retinopathy

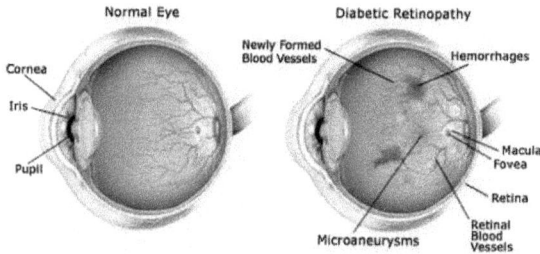

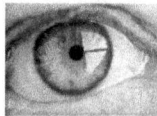

Normal Eye

Diabetic Retinopathy

Newly Formed
Blood Vessels

Hemorrhages

Cornea

Iris

Pupil

Macula
Fovea

Retina

Retinal
Blood
Vessels

Microaneurysms

DID YOU KNOW???

Getting your annual eye exam can
detect early symptoms of diabetes,
high blood pressure, shingles,
tumors, stroke, high cholesterol,
hypertension, arthritis, HIV... and
that's just to name a few.

Your eye are the windows to your health!

(16) DIABETIC AUTONOMIC NEUROPATHY (DAN) - ANSITEST BY ANSISCOPE:

Autonomic neuropathy alludes to harm to the autonomic nerves. This harm upsets flags between the mind and segments of the autonomic sensory system, for example, the heart, veins and sweat organs. This can cause a diminished or irregular presentation of at least one automatic body capacities.

Indications:

Signs and indications of autonomic neuropathy shift, contingent upon which some portion of your autonomic sensory system is influenced. They may incorporate

- ✓ Sluggish understudy response - Making it hard to change from light to dim and causing issues with driving around evening time.
- ✓ Silent myocardial ischemia or cardiovascular denervation disorder (Cardiac Autonomic Neuropathy - CAN) - Rhythm aggravation in the heart, prompting extremely fast pulses (Fibrillation).
- ✓ Dizziness and blacking out - after standing brought about by a drop in pulse.
- ✓ Difficulty in processing nourishment - Due to unusual stomach related capacity and moderate purging of the stomach (gastroparesis). This can cause a sentiment of completion subsequent to eating even a little amount of nourishment, loss of hunger, the runs, clogging, stomach swelling, sickness, heaving and acid reflux.
- ✓ Impaired Salivary organ brokenness - Causing diminished salivary emission prompting gum contamination and awful stench in the mouth.
- ✓ Sweating variations from the norm - Such as inordinate or diminished perspiring, which influences the capacity to manage internal heat level. Exorbitant perspiring might be uneven and may happen while taking nourishment.
- ✓ Urinary issues - Including trouble in beginning pee, direness, recurrence and a powerlessness to purge your bladder, which can prompt urinary tract diseases.
- ✓ Sexual brokenness - Including issues accomplishing or keeping up an erection (erectile brokenness) or discharge issues in men. Vaginal dryness, troubles with excitement and climax in ladies.

Ineffectively controlled diabetes builds the danger of creating autonomic neuropathy. The hazard is more noteworthy for individuals who have had diabetes for a long time and experience issues controlling their glucose. Also, individuals with diabetes who are overweight, have hypertension, elevated cholesterol has a higher danger of autonomic neuropathy.

Analysis:

ANSITEST assists with estimating the brokenness of this autonomic framework as indicated by your age which keeps you from major issues as referenced previously.

ANSISCOPE is utilized to perform ANSITEST which is a safe and non-intrusive test for checking the autonomic sensory system. It takes 5 to 10 minutes to finish the test with no pinprick or agony.

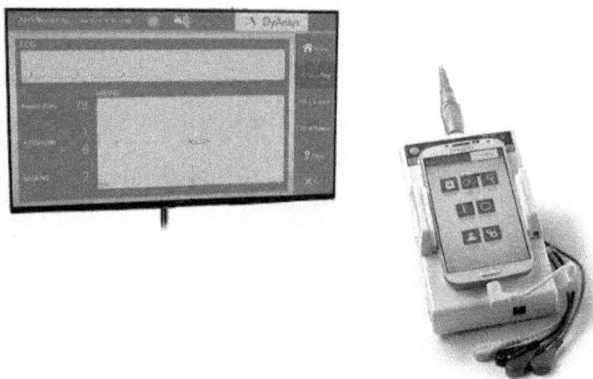

ANSISCOPE

9. PREVENTION AND TREATMENT OF DIABETES

OBJECTIVES OF TREATMENT OF DIABETES:

The patient ought to

- ✓ Attain and keep up suitable body weight.
- ✓ Keep his glucose and fat levels in the blood inside as far as possible
- ✓ Have normal registration.
- ✓ Be kept away from or treated from the symptoms of the medication.
- ✓ Learn to live inside the breaking points of the infection.
- ✓ Be alleviated of practically all the side effects.
- ✓ Be ready to lead a typical or close ordinary life in the public arena.

PREVENTION AND TREATMENT OF DIABETES TYPE 1 AND TYPE 2:

Below is a list of the current methods used to treat diabetes type 1 and type 2:

	Diabetes type 1	Diabetes type 2
Cure	None. A few scientists are as of now taking a gander at the potential advantages of a mix of immunosuppressant medications and medications that expansion gastrin generation to support pancreatic recovery that may permit individuals with type 1 diabetes to live insulin-free.	There is no remedy for type 2 diabetes, albeit some of the time gastric medical procedure, way of life and prescription treatment can bring about abatement. Physical exercise, sound loss of weight and diet control is exhorted.
Treatment	• Injections of insulin • Oral meds (less normal) • Dietary adjustments	• Using diabetes medicines • Sometimes insulin injections • Sometimes insulin infusions • Healthy nourishment decisions • Self Monitoring of Blood Glucose (SMBG)

		Controlling circulatory strain
	modifications	• Controlling circulatory strain
	• Physically movement	• Monitoring cholesterol levels.
	• Regular registration of glucose levels	.
	• Controlling circulatory strain	
	• Monitoring cholesterol levels.	
Prevention	• No realized approach to forestall the loss of pancreatic, insulin-delivering cells.	• Preventable and can be deferred with a sound eating regimen and exercise.

Different treatment for diabetes is talked about under the accompanying headings:

1. Diabetes Dietary administration

    ✓ Diabetes Nutrition
    ✓ Diabetes Diet
    ✓ Diabetes Food Groups
    ✓ Diabetes Drinks
    ✓ Diabetes Sweeteners

2. Physical exercise

3. Yoga

4. Care - Meditation

5. Pressure point massage

6. Needle therapy

7. Back rub treatment and Reflexology

8. Fragrance based treatment

9. Music treatment

10. Biofeedback

11. Ayurvedic natural prescription

12. Homeopathy

13. Allopathy

- ✓ Oral drugs
- ✓ Insulin (pen/infusion)
- ✓ Insulin siphons
- ✓ One of the propelled treatment for neuropathy is INFRARED LIGHT THERAPY
- ✓ Treatment for Chronic Hyperglycemia related with irresistible sicknesses.

10. DIABETES DIETARY MANAGEMENT
DIABETES NUTRITION

YOU DON'T HAVE TO EAT LESS, YOU IMMEDIATELY INCLUDE TO EAT RIGHT

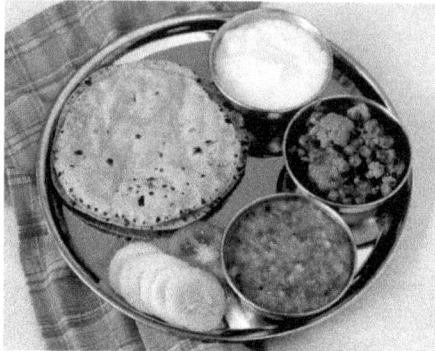

Compelling administration of diabetes can be accomplished with a proper eating regimen. Patients with recently analyzed diabetes ought to get counsel from a dietitian not long after analysis.

Sustenance is a basic piece of diabetes care. Adjusting the perfect measure of starches, fat, protein alongside fiber, nutrients and minerals causes us to keep up a solid eating routine and a sound way of life. The nutrition classes that give nourishment can be isolated into two as

✓ Macronutrients
✓ Micronutrients

MACRONUTRIENTS:

The three nutrition types that give us vitality to be specific: starches, fat and protein. These three significant supplements are the suppliers of fuel for our bodies.

Carbohydrate:

Sugar is one of the body's fundamental wellsprings of vitality. Starch is separated into glucose generally rapidly and subsequently has a more articulated impact on glucose levels than either fat or protein. Sugar is found in a wide assortment of nourishment, prominently in dull nourishments, for example, rice, pasta and flour (along these lines including baked good,

84

bread and other batter based nourishments). Sugar is additionally a type of starch. Starch is commonly found in all foods grown from the ground. Foods grown from the ground with generally high starch content incorporate Potatoes, Root vegetables (Carrot, Beetroot), Mangoes, Bananas and Pears.

Sorts of Carbohydrate:

There are various sorts of sugar which are separated rapidly or less rapidly due to their concoction structure.

Basic starches are sugars that are separated rapidly by the body and along these lines raise glucose levels rapidly. Sugars are found in an assortment of normal nourishment sources including organic product, vegetables and milk and give nourishment a sweet taste. Be that as it may, they likewise raise blood glucose levels rapidly. Sugars can be classified as single sugars (monosaccharides) which incorporate glucose, fructose and galactose or twofold sugars (disaccharides) which incorporate sucrose (table sugar), lactose and maltose.

The National Health Service (NHS) encourages grown-ups to expend under 70g per day of sugar for men and under 50g of sugar a day for ladies. Notwithstanding, individuals with diabetes will profit by better blood glucose levels if sugar admission can be constrained to bring down levels.

Complex sugars are starches that are separated more gradually than straightforward sugars and will raise sugar levels all the more gradually. Complex sugars, otherwise called polysaccharides framed by longer saccharide chains which implies they take more time to separate. They incorporate white bread, cakes and baked goods.

Proposal of the Scientific Advisory Committee on Nutrition (SACN):

Starch legitimately impacts glucose levels and it is essential to know about how much sugar you are having at every supper. It is frequently simple to think little of precisely how much sugar you are having, especially when eating boring nourishments, for example, pasta, rice and potatoes.

The SACN prescribes that half of our every day vitality originates from starches. This adds up to around 225 to 300g of sugars for individuals on an eating routine of 2,000 to 2,500 calories. The proposals are ordinarily passed down to patients through the NHS.

Fat:

Fat is one of the fundamental macronutrients. Fat is required by the body for giving vitality, keeping hair and skin sound, helping our cells to work appropriately and for ensuring our body and organs. It doesn't straightforwardly raise our glucose levels whether we have diabetes or not. Fats are found in a scope of nourishments which incorporate nuts, avocados, beans, fish, meat, milk, cheddar and other dairy items. Fat is additionally utilized in the singing of nourishments and inside handled food sources including crisps, cakes, baked goods and other bread kitchen food sources.

Unsaturated fats:

Unsaturated fats that are found in nuts, avocados, slick fish, and oils, for example, sunflower and olive oil. They are frequently alluded to as 'great fats'.

Soaked fats:

They are much of the time found in less solid nourishments, for example, crisps, chips and biscuits however they are additionally found in meats, margarine and another dairy.

Proposal of the Scientific Advisory Committee on Nutrition (SACN):

The proposals are commonly passed down to patients through the NHS. The counsel of the NHS is for individuals to decrease the measure of fat and especially soaked fat in their eating routine. The low-fat methodology has been unequivocally suggested for individuals with diabetes.

Fibre:

Dietary fiber is otherwise called roughage. It is the general term for a scope of various sugars found in the eating routine which are not processed by the body.

Kinds of Fiber:

Filaments which break up in warm water. Dissolvable fiber ties with water to shape a gel and this has been appeared to have advantageous properties in hindering assimilation and the retention of vitality from the nourishment. The manner in which solvent fiber acts has benefits for bringing down cholesterol, improving blood glucose levels, diminishing craving and improving heart wellbeing.

Insoluble fiber:

Filaments which don't break up in warm water. They assume a fundamental job in helping matter to travel through the gut productively, assisting with diminishing entrail issues, for example, stoppage, hemorrhoids and diverticulosis.

Proposal of SACN:

The NHS takes note of that the normal individual just has 14g of fiber day by day. The Department of Health suggests that the majority of us ought to have 18g of fiber daily. The NHS suggests expanding fiber steadily as unexpected increments in fiber could prompt stomach squeezes and swelling for the time being. On the off chance that expanding your day by day fiber consumption, guarantee you keep yourself hydrated. It is prescribed to have around 1.2 liters of liquid daily which is around 6-8 mugs or glasses a day.

Protein:

It is one of the macronutrients. It encourages the body to develop new tissue, in this manner assisting with building muscle and fix harm to the body. Protein can be separated into glucose by the body and utilized for vitality (a procedure known as gluconeogenesis).

Protein is separated into glucose less proficiently than starch and therefore, any impacts of protein on blood glucose levels will in general happen anyplace between a couple of hours and a few hours subsequent to eating.

While taking a generally protein-based dinner, individuals with type 1diabetes or type 2 diabetes on insulin, should bear the impacts of protein at the top of the priority list.

Proposal:

- ✓ 1 to 3 years: 15g
- ✓ 4 to 6 years: 20g
- ✓ 7 to 10 years: 28g
- ✓ 11 to 14 years: 42g
- ✓ 15 to 18 years: 55g
- ✓ 19 to 50 years: 55g

✓ More than 50 years: 53g

Protein and Cancer:

The examinations found that nonstop utilization of handled red meat builds the odds of creating sicknesses, for example, lung disease, liver malignant growth and eminently entrail disease. Having a specific abundance of protein in the eating routine, especially in blend with liquor might prompt issues, for example, gout.

Salt:

Salt is viewed as a much-esteemed mineral. Admission of salt is essential for the human body and aides in directing water levels in the body, keeping up typical pH of blood and transmission of nerve signals. The mineral can't be created by the body yet it gets discharged implies that standard admission of salt is important. Numerous nourishments fill in as a wellspring of salt. Nourishments that are high in salt incorporate Ready dinners, soup, bread, breakfast grain, pre-made sauces –, for example, pasta sauces, pizza, pies and cakes, cheddar, sauce granules, bacon, prawns and salted fish.

Suggestion:

The Department of Health suggests that every individual doesn't take more than 6g of salt a day, which is proportionate to one teaspoon of salt over the day.

A few nourishments will state how a lot of sodium is in nourishment instead of saying how much salt. In the event that the bundling cites the measure of sodium, this should be increased by 2.5 to get the equal measure of salt.

Salt and High Blood Pressure:

Salt has been connected with raised pulse levels. The investigations demonstrated that a low sodium diet diminished normal circulatory strain levels. Hypertension is connected with multiple times higher danger of coronary illness and stroke. Hypertension in diabetic individuals gets an opportunity of an expansion in the danger of microvascular difficulties, for example, retinopathy, nephropathy (kidney sickness) and neuropathy (nerve harm).

MICRONUTRIENTS:

Micronutrients incorporate all nutrients and minerals that we take it in and are a basic piece of a diabetic eating routine.

Dietary Supplements:

Dietary enhancements are items that can assist us with getting the correct parity of significant supplements in our every day consumes less calories. They are otherwise called a nourishment supplement or wholesome enhancement.

Different inquires about have demonstrated that specific nutrients, minerals, herbs and flavors can help with overseeing diabetes and at times treat or forestall diabetes-related complexities, for example, neuropathy (nerve harm). Some have likewise been appeared to lessen the danger of creating type 2 diabetes.

The significant dietary enhancements incorporate Alpha-lipoic corrosive (ALA), Chromium, Coenzyme Q10, Vitamin D, Magnesium, Potassium and Zinc, Polycystic Ovary Syndrome. There is some proof that herbs, flavors and other plant-based enhancements are recommended which can support diabetic patients. These incorporate Aloe Vera, Bitter melon, Cinnamon, Fenugreek and Ginger.

(1)   Alpha-lipoic corrosive (ALA):

It is a nutrient like synthetic called a cancer prevention agent.

SOURCES:

Yeast, Spinach, Broccoli and Potatoes.

Capacity:

They help to forestall specific sorts of cell harm in the body and furthermore reestablishes nutrient levels, for example, Vitamin E and C. They can likewise improve the capacity and conduction of neurons in diabetes. It is utilized in the body to separate starches and to make vitality for different organs in the body. It may secure the cerebrum under states of harm or damage. The cancer prevention agent impacts may likewise be useful in certain liver sicknesses.

Employments:

✓ To treat nerve-related manifestations of diabetes:

Consuming, torment and deadness in the legs and arms.

✓ To treat eye-related issue of diabetes:

Harm to the retina, waterfalls, glaucoma and an eye sickness called Wilson's illness.

✓ To treat constant weariness disorder (CFS), memory misfortune and Lyme sickness.

Dosages:

The logical research recommended 600 to 1200 mg every day for treating type 2 diabetes and to improve side effects, for example, consuming, agony and deadness in the legs.

(2) Gamma-linolenic corrosive (GLA):

It is an omega-6 unsaturated fat (greasy substance) found in different plant seed oils.

SOURCES:

Borage oil (got from the seeds of the Borago officinalis) and evening primrose oil (Oenothera biennis), blackcurrant (Ribes nigrum) seed oil and hemp seed oil (got from hemp seeds).

Capacity:

It is an omega-6 unsaturated fat, which the body can change over to substances that diminish aggravation and cell development.

Employments:

Taking gamma-linolenic corrosive by mouth for 6 a year appears to diminish side effects and forestall nerve harm in individuals with nerve torment because of type 1 or type 2 diabetes. Gamma-linolenic corrosive appears to work better in individuals with great glucose control.

Gamma-linolenic corrosive (GLA) is additionally utilized for conditions that influence the skin including fundamental sclerosis, psoriasis and dermatitis. It is additionally utilized for rheumatoid arthritis(RA), polyps in the mouth, elevated cholesterol and other blood fats, coronary illness, metabolic disorder (Syndrome-X), diabetic nerve torment, consideration shortage hyperactivity issue (ADHD), despondency, misery after childbirth, interminable weariness disorder (CFS), and roughage fever (unfavorably susceptible rhinitis). A few people use it to forestall disease and to help bosom malignant growth patients react quicker to treatment with the medication tamoxifen.

Dosages:

The logical research recommended 360 to 480 mg every day for treating diabetic nerve torment.

(3) Chromium:

It is a metal and a basic follow component. It is essential in a self-effacing quantity for human wellbeing.

SOURCES:

Broccoli (53%), Barley (23%), Oats (15%), Green Beans (6%), Tomatoes (4%), Romaine Lettuce (4%) and Black Pepper (3%)

Capacity:

Chromium may assist with keeping glucose levels ordinary by improving the manner in which our bodies use insulin.

Employments:

It is utilized for controlling high glucose levels in individuals with prediabetes, type 1 and type 2 diabetes. Taking Chromium picolinate (a synthetic intensify that contains chromium) by mouth brings down high glucose and assists insulin with working in individuals with type 2 diabetes. Likewise, chromium picolinate may diminish weight increase and fat collection in individuals with type 2 diabetes who are taking one of the doctor prescribed medications called sulfonylureas.

It is likewise utilized for gloom, polycystic ovary disorder (PCOS), bringing down "awful" cholesterol (LDL), and raising "great" cholesterol (HDL).

Portions:

Type 2 diabetes – 200 to 1000 mcg day by day in partitioned portions.

Cholesterol – 15 to 200 mcg day by day for 7 to 16 months brings down triglycerides and low-thickness lipoprotein (LDL), and builds high – thickness lipoprotein (HDL).

In 2001, the National Academy of Sciences distributed Dietary Reference Intakes (DRI) for chromium. These DRI suggestions came as Adequate Intake (AI) levels as follows:

- ✓ 0 a half year: 0.2 mcg
- ✓ 6 months-1 year: 5.5 mcg
- ✓ 1-3 years: 11 mcg
- ✓ 4-8 years: 15 mcg
- ✓ 9-13 years, female: 21 mcg
- ✓ 9-13 years, male, 25 mcg
- ✓ 14-18 years, female: 24 mcg
- ✓ 14-18 years, male: 35 mcg
- ✓ 19-50 years, female: 25 mcg
- ✓ 19-50 years, male: 35 mcg
- ✓ 51+ years, female: 20 mcg
- ✓ 51+ years, male: 30 mcg
- ✓ Pregnant ladies, 14-18 years: 29 mcg
- ✓ Pregnant ladies, 19+ years: 30 mcg
- ✓ Lactating ladies, 14-18 years: 44 mcg
- ✓ Lactating ladies, 19+ years: 45 mcg

(4) Coenzyme Q10 (CoQ10):

It is a supplement that happens normally in the body. It goes about as a cancer prevention agent, which shields cells from harm and has a significant impact in the digestion. It is otherwise called Q10, nutrient Q10, ubiquinone or ubidecarenone.

SOURCES:

Broccoli, Spinach, Cauliflower, Orange, Strawberries, Fish, Beef, Chicken, Peanuts, Sesame seeds, Soybean oil and Canola oil.

Capacity:

Coenzymes assist catalysts with attempting to process nourishment and perform other body procedures, and they help secure the heart and skeletal muscles.

Employments:

It can bring down circulatory strain marginally. CoQ10 is likewise used to treat cardiovascular breakdown and other heart conditions, conceivably assisting with improving a few side effects and decrease future cardiovascular dangers.

Portions:

50 milligrams to 1,200 milligrams in grown-ups split into a few portions for every day.

(5) Vitamin D:

It is a fat-solvent nutrient that assumes a significant job in keeping up the soundness of bones, teeth, joints and aiding insusceptible framework work.

SOURCES:

It is found in specific nourishments but on the other hand is created by the body because of introduction to the sun. The principle source is the sun's bright B (UVB) beams.

Capacity:

At the point when the sun's bright B (UVB) beams are presented to uncovered skin, the body changes over a cholesterol subordinate into Vitamin D. Each cell and tissue inside the body has a Vitamin D protein receptor.

TYPES:

✓ Vitamin D2 (Ergocalciferol) – Synthetic rendition which has a shorter time span of usability.

✓ Vitamin D3 (Cholecalciferol) – It is equivalent to the Vitamin D created by the body following introduction to UVB beams. It is multiple occasions as powerful as nutrient D2

Employments:

Nutrient D assists with improving the body's affectability to insulin and in this way lessen the danger of insulin opposition, which is frequently a forerunner to type 2 diabetes. It might assist with managing the generation of insulin in the pancreas.

It assists with decreasing parathyroid hormone (PTH) levels, which in the long haul may advance weight reduction and diminish the danger of heftiness, which is a significant hazard factor for type 2 diabetes. Nutrient D can build a person's body's degrees of the hormone leptin, which controls muscle to fat ratio stockpiling and triggers the vibe of having eaten enough and therefore bringing down craving levels. It can help lower levels of Cortisol, a pressure hormone created in the adrenal organs. The expansion in the hormone in the blood prompts stomach fat which is connected to different wellbeing conditions including diabetes type 2.

Portions:

The day by day measurement of 400 International Units (IU).

Nutrient D levels of an individual ought to preferably be between 20-56 ng/ml (50-140 nmol/l). The right degree of Vitamin D fluctuates from individual to individual.

11. POLYCYSTIC OVARY SYNDROME

Polycystic ovary disorder (PCOS) is one of the most well-known endocrine issue as often as possible portrayed by the aggregation of various growths (liquid filled sacs) on the ovaries related with high male hormone levels (hyperandrogenism), ovulatory brokenness, stomach stoutness, and other metabolic unsettling influences. At first called the Stein and Leventhal disorder after its disclosure during the 1935s, the term additionally manages multisystem inclusion including hyperinsulinism, hyperlipidemia, expanded androgens, endometrial hyperplasia, diabetes mellitus, stoutness, anovulation, heart illness and fruitlessness.

TWO MAIN TYPES OF PCOS

1. Insulin-Resistant PCOS

Insulin-Resistant PCOS is additionally alluded to as Type 1 PCOS, and it is frequently connected with the exemplary indications of PCOS. These incorporate weight gain, ovulatory interferences, facial hair, male pattern baldness and skin inflammation. Those with Insulin-Resistant PCOS additionally show a more prominent potential for creating diabetes and expanded testosterone levels the two of which are brought about by the hidden insulin obstruction. Insulin obstruction changes the hypothalamic-pituitary-ovarian pivot prompts incitement of theca cell to create the overabundance measure of androgen and decrease in the degree of SHBG amalgamation in liver cells bringing about hyperandrogenism and anovulation prompts the polycystic ovarian disorder.

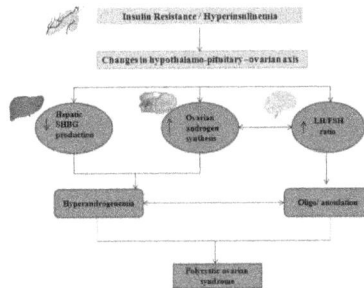

Insulin Resistant Polycystic ovary syndrome

2. Non-Insulin Resistant PCOS

Right now PCOS brought about by Vitamin D or Iodine lack, hormone-upsetting poisons, thyroid infection, and adrenal pressure. For ladies encountering Non-Insulin Resistant PCOS, hostile to Diabetic medications won't influence the condition, and neither one of the wills help in decreasing the weight which is increased because of hormonal unevenness. The treatment choices, right now, to being progressively normal. Patients might be impacted to stay away from dairy while likewise being endorsed enhancements, for example, Iodine, Vitamin D, Magnesium, and Zinc, alongside natural equations to decrease testosterone. Regular progesterone may likewise be endorsed to improve the hormonal irregularity and incite ovulation.

The study of disease transmission OF PCOS:

In the United States, polycystic ovarian disorder (PCOS) is one of the most well-known endocrine issue of regenerative age ladies, with a pervasiveness of 4-12%. Up to 10% of ladies are determined to have PCOS during gynecologic visits. In some European investigations, the pervasiveness of PCOS has been accounted for to be 6.5-8%. A lot of ethnic fluctuation in hirsutism is watched. For instance, Asian (East and Southeast Asia) ladies have less hirsutism than white ladies given a similar serum androgen esteems. In an examination that evaluated hirsutism in southern Chinese ladies, specialists found a predominance of 10.5%. In hirsute ladies, there was a noteworthy increment in the occurrence of skin inflammation, menstrual inconsistencies, polycystic ovaries, and acanthosis nigricans.

PCOS influences premenopausal ladies, and the period of beginning is regularly perimenarchal (before bone age arrives at 16 y). Be that as it may, clinical acknowledgment of the disorder might be postponed by the disappointment of the patient to get worried by unpredictable menses, hirsutism, or different side effects or by the cover of PCOS discoveries with typical physiologic development during the 2 years after menarche. In lean ladies with a hereditary inclination to PCOS, the disorder might be exposed when they in this manner put on weight. The predominance of hirsutism, skin break out, female example male pattern baldness, acanthosis nigricans, seborrhea, striae, and acrochordons was seen as 78%, 48%, 31%, 30%, 29%, 13%, and 9%, separately.

PATHOGENESIS

Pathogenesis is unpredictable and not entirely comprehended. At the point when insulin discharge can never again remunerate the insulin obstruction, hyperglycemia creates. Insulin obstruction is it's trademark. Proof exists for beta-cell brokenness and impeded insulin discharge in individuals with type 2 DM and those in danger of it. It likewise incorporates the debilitated first-stage insulin emission because of IV glucose imbuement, lost ordinarily pulsatile insulin discharge, an expansion in proinsulin emission flagging, weakened insulin preparing, and amassing of islet amyloid polypeptide (a protein typically emitted with insulin). High glucose levels desensitize beta cells and cause beta-cell brokenness (glucose harmfulness), or both and the insulin discharge is weakened by Hyperglycaemia. Within the sight of insulin obstruction, it takes a long time to build up these changes.

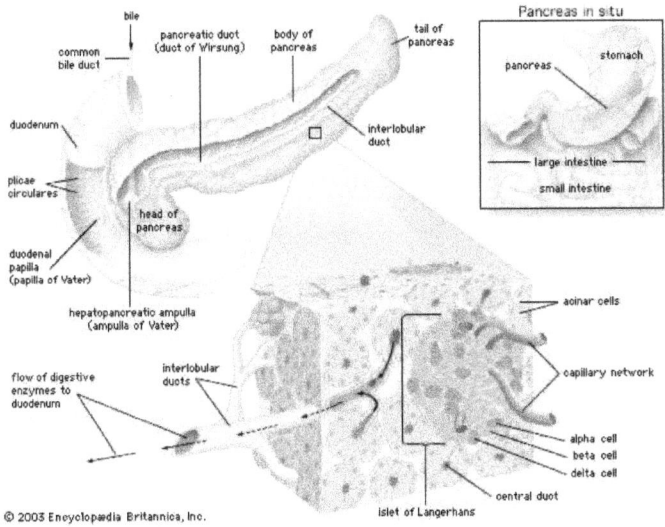

Representative diagram of pathogenesis of diabetes mellitus

PATHOGENESIS AND RISK FACTORS OF PCOS

1. Hereditary qualities: PCOS is accepted to be a mind boggling jumble, with hereditary just as natural elements adding to the improvement of the ailment. 20-40% of female first-degree family members of ladies with PCOS additionally have the disorder, proposing that the illness is incompletely heritable and groups in families.

2. Intrauterine exposures: exposures to testosterone in utero may incline to the later advancement of PCOS. Creature considers have shown that in utero introduction is related

with the improvement of a PCOS-like disorder including hyperinsulinemia, hyperandrogenism, oligoanovulation, and polycystic ovaries.

3. Condition/way of life: a few way of life factors and natural exposures have been related with a progressively extreme PCOS phenotype. An inactive way of life is related with expanded metabolic brokenness, and weight gain is related with oligoanovulation and hyperandrogenism.

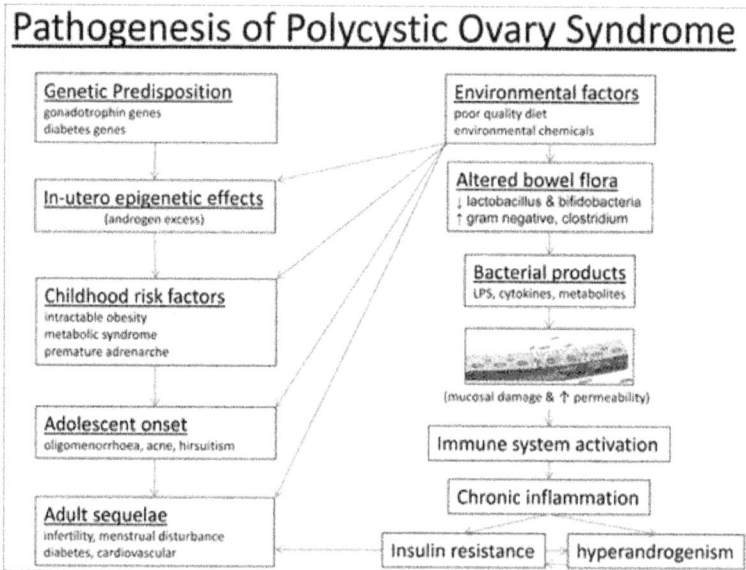

Pathogenesis of Polycystic Ovary Syndrome

4. **Corpulence:** in spite of the fact that weight isn't accepted to cause PCOS, it is known to compound the side effects of the malady. Stoutness is available in 30-75% of ladies with PCOS.

CONTRAST BETWEEN NORMAL MENSTRUAL CYCLE AND POLYCYSTIC OVARIAN SYNDROME MENSTRUAL CYCLE

1. Typical Menstrual Cycles

The menstrual cycle begins when the mind sends LH and FSH to the ovaries. A major flood of LH is the sign that makes the ovaries ovulate, or discharge an egg. The egg goes down the fallopian tube and into the uterus. Progesterone from the ovary makes the covering of the uterus thicken. In the event that the egg isn't treated the covering of the uterus is shed. This is a menstrual period. After the menstrual period, the cycle starts once more. The graph right side shows a normal menstrual cycle, and the chart on the left side shows a PCOS cycle with no ovulation.

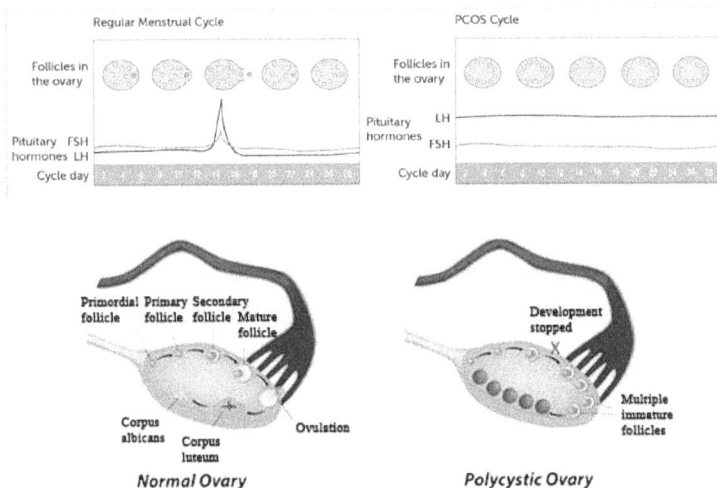

Difference between Normal Menstrual Cycle and PCOS Menstrual Cycle

Menstrual cycle in PCOS

In ladies with polycystic ovary disorder (PCOS), numerous little follicles (little pimples 4 to 9 mm in dm) gather in the ovary, thus the term polycystic ovaries. None of these little follicles are fit for developing to a size that would trigger ovulation. Thus, the degrees of estrogen, progesterone, LH, and FSH become imbalanced. Androgens are typically created by the ovaries and the adrenal organs. Instances of androgens incorporate testosterone, androstenedione, dehydroepiandrosterone (DHEA), and DHEA sulfate (DHEAS). Androgens may get expanded in ladies with PCOS in view of the significant levels of LH yet in addition due to elevated levels of insulin that are generally observed with PCOS.

PCOS Etiology

1. Insulin Resistance

Insulin is a hormone delivered by the pancreas to control the measure of sugar in the blood. It assists with moving glucose from the blood into cells, where it's separated to deliver vitality. Insulin obstruction implies the body's tissues are impervious with the impacts of insulin. Elevated levels of insulin cause the ovaries to deliver an excess of testosterone, which meddles with the advancement of the follicles and forestalls ordinary ovulation. Insulin opposition can likewise prompt weight gain. Insulin obstruction is a pathophysiological patron in around half to 80% of ladies with PCOS, particularly in overweight ladies. On the other hand, lean ladies and ladies with milder PCOS seem to have less extreme hyperinsulinemia and insulin opposition. Insulin opposition adds to metabolic highlights yet additionally regenerative highlights through expanding androgen creation and expanding free androgens by decreasing sex hormone-restricting globulin (SHBG).

Schema of aetiology and features of PCOS

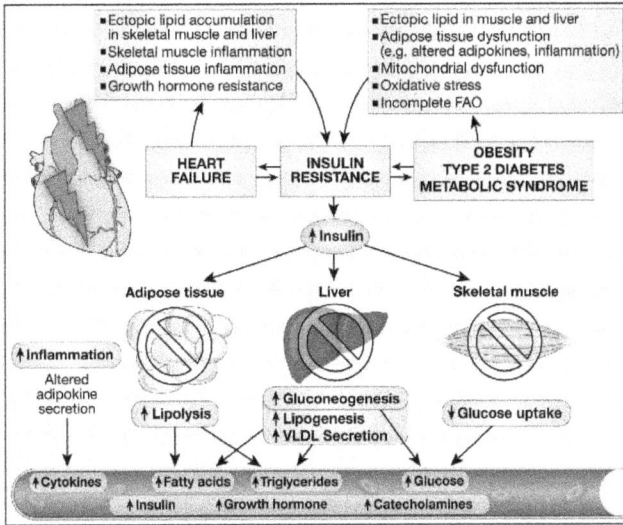

- Ectopic lipid accumulation in skeletal muscle and liver
- Skeletal muscle inflammation
- Adipose tissue inflammation
- Growth hormone resistance

- Ectopic lipid in muscle and liver
- Adipose tissue dysfunction (e.g. altered adipokines, inflammation)
- Mitochondrial dysfunction
- Oxidative stress
- Incomplete FAO

HEART FAILURE ↔ **INSULIN RESISTANCE** ↔ **OBESITY TYPE 2 DIABETES METABOLIC SYNDROME**

↑Insulin

Adipose tissue   Liver   Skeletal muscle

↑Inflammation
Altered adipokine secretion

↑Lipolysis

↑Gluconeogenesis
↑Lipogenesis
↑VLDL Secretion

↓Glucose uptake

↑Cytokines   ↑Fatty acids   ↑Triglycerides   ↓Glucose
↑Insulin   ↑Growth hormone   ↑Catecholamines

101

Outline of components that lead to insulin opposition in cardiovascular breakdown or metabolic disorder. Flagging occasions in skeletal muscle, liver and fat tissue. Signs and Symptoms of Insulin Resistance, Insulin obstruction is normally disturbed by a blend of components connected to weight, age, hereditary qualities, being stationary and smoking, An enormous midsection , The most ideal approach to tell whether the individual is in danger for insulin opposition is by estimating the midriff. An abdomen that estimates 35 inches or more for ladies, at least 40 for men, is progressively inclined to insulin obstruction. Notwithstanding an enormous midsection, on the off chance that there are at least three of the accompanying, at that point the individual is probably going to have metabolic disorder, which makes insulin obstruction. High triglycerides , Those having cholesterol levels of 150 or higher. , On the off chance that the Low-thickness lipoprotein level is beneath 50 for ladies and 40 or men – or taking medicine to raise low high-thickness lipoprotein (HDL) levels. Low HDLs , High glucose , On the off chance that the glucose level is of 100-125 mg/dl (the prediabetes go) or more than 125 (diabetes). , High fasting glucose, On the off chance that the individual is on medication to treat high glucose. Mellow high glucose might be an early indication of diabetes. Dark skin patches There might be unmistakable skin changes in the event of serious insulin opposition. This is spoken to by patches of obscured skin on the rear of the neck or elbows, knees, knuckles or armpits. This staining is called acanthosis nigricans. There is a high danger of cardiovascular ailment in individuals with insulin opposition, prediabetes and type 2 diabetes. As per the International Diabetes Federation insulin opposition pairs the hazard for coronary failure and stroke – and significantly increases the hazard for respiratory failure or 'cerebrum assault' which will be savage.

2. Hormone irregularity Numerous ladies with PCOS are found to have an irregularity in specific hormones. It incorporates.

- ✓ Raised levels of testosterone (T) – a hormone regularly thought of as a male hormone, albeit all ladies for the most part produce limited quantities of it.
- ✓ Raised levels of Luteinizing hormone (LH) – this animates ovulation yet may abnormally affect the ovaries if levels are excessively high. Low degrees of sex hormone-restricting globulin (SHBG) – a protein in the blood, which ties to testosterone and decreases its impact.
- ✓ Raised levels of Prolactin–a hormone that invigorates the bosom organs to create milk in pregnancy (just in certain ladies with PCOS)

3. Hereditary qualities

PCOS is a multifactorial infection that occasionally runs in families. On the off chance that any family members, for example, your mom, sister or auntie, have PCOS, at that point the danger of creating it is frequently expanded. This recommends there might be a hereditary connect to PCOS, albeit explicit qualities related with the condition are still under research.

CLINICAL FEATURES OF PCOS

Ladies with PCOS may give an assortment of clinical end results including:

- ✓ Reproductive indications like Menstrual inconsistencies, Hirsutism, Infertility and Pregnancy complexities
- ✓ Metabolic suggestions like Insulin opposition, Obesity, Metabolic disorder, IGT, DM2 and Potentially CVD
- ✓ Psychological issues incorporate diminished personal satisfaction, poor confidence, despondency, nervousness, and so forth. Clinical indications of PCOS.

Highlights of PCOS may show at any age, extending from youth (untimely pubescence), adolescent (Hirsutism, Menstrual inconsistencies), early adulthood and center life (fruitlessness, Glucose bigotry) in later life (Diabetes Mellitus and Cardiovascular malady).

Manifestations of Ovarian dysfunction	Manifestations of Hyperandrogenism	Associated conditions
Oligomenorrhea	Hirsutism	Obesity
Amenorrhea	Acne	Insulin resistance
USG-Polycystic	Alopecia	Impaired fasting glucose
ovaries	Seborrhea	Type 2 diabetes mellitus
	Acanthosis Nigricans	Dyslipidemia
	(Excess Circulating antigens)	Metabolic syndrome
		Mood disorders
		Arterial hypertension

Clinical manifestations and associated conditions

Reproductive Manifestations of PCOS

Ovarian brokenness

Ovarian brokenness typically shows as oligomenorrhoea/amenorrhoea coming about because of constant oligo-ovulation/anovulation. In any case, delayed anovulation can prompt useless uterine draining which may imitate progressively normal menstrual cycles. Most of PCOS patients have ovarian brokenness, with 70% to 80% of ladies with PCOS giving oligomenorrhoea or amenorrhoea. Oligomenorrhoea happens for the most part in pre-adulthood, with beginning further down the road regularly connected with weight gain. Menorrhagia can happen with unopposed estrogen and endometrial hyperplasia, further exacerbated by raised estrogen levels in heftiness.

Barrenness

It is the most well-known reason for anovulatory fruitlessness. It represents 90% to 95% of ladies going to fruitlessness centers with anovulation. Notwithstanding, 60% of ladies with PCOS are rich, in spite of the fact that opportunity to imagine is regularly expanded. Heftiness autonomously fuels barrenness and incites a more serious danger of premature delivery.

Hyperandrogenism

The clinical and biochemical indications of androgen abundance in PCOS result from expanded blend and arrival of ovarian androgens. Clinical hyperandrogenism principally incorporates Hirsutism, Acne and seborrhea and Male example alopecia.

Hirsutism

PCOS is a typical reason for hirsutism happening in around 60% of cases; notwithstanding, this shifts with race and level of heftiness. Hirsutism is characterized as the nearness of over the top terminal hair in zones of the body that are androgens-subordinate and typically bare or with restricted hair development, for example, the face, upper lip, jaw chest, guts, back, areolas, thighs and arms. It alludes to a male example of body hair (androgenic hair). Regularly, in females after pubarche, the major androgenic atoms are Dehydroepiandrosterone sulfate (DHEAS), Androstenedione, Dehydroepiandrostenedione, Testosterone, and Dihydrotestosterone (DHT), in plunging request of serum focus.

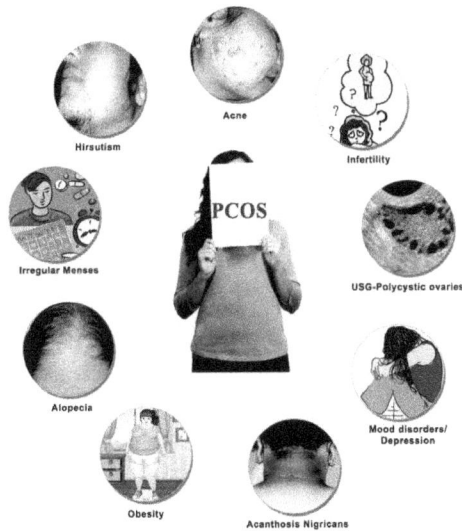

Clinical manifestations of PCOS

12. DIABETES DIET

"DIABETES NUTRIENTS EAT TO LIVE AND NOT LIVE TO EAT"

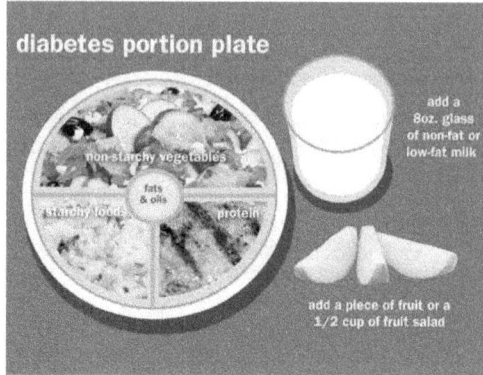

Nutritionists and Dieticians arranged the diabetic eating routine into two to be specific

(1)   Measured diabetic eating routine

(2)   Unmeasured diabetic eating routine

ESTIMATED DIABETIC DIET:

The specific amounts of staples to be taken are said something this kind of diet. This is significant for some moderately aged stout diabetics who need to get more fit to control diabetes. Unhealthy staples ought to be weighed at first and taken with legitimate consideration. Later they can judge precisely even without gauging.

MEASURED DIET CHART (1500 Kcal):

Morning Bed Tea:

✓ 1 cup tea or espresso (milk 30 ml without sugar).

Breakfast:

✓ 1 egg or paneer 30 gm.

✓ 1 cut bread or 2 chapattis (20 gm) or idli.

✓ 1 cup milk (30 ml without sugar).

Early in the day snacks:

✓ 4 salted scones or 1 organic product.

✓ 1 cup of tea or espresso (30 ml milk without sugar).

Lunch:

✓ Dal (30 gm) or paneer (35 gm) or lamb (50 gm) or chicken (70 gm) or fish (100 gm).
✓ 2 chapattis (20 gm).
✓ Blended vegetables (100 gm).
✓ Curd (120 gm) or buttermilk.
✓ Plate of mixed greens (125 gm).

Night Tea:

✓ 4 salted rolls or 1 natural product.
✓ 1 cup of tea or espresso (30 ml milk without sugar).

Supper:

✓ Dal (30 gm) or paneer (35 gm) or lamb (50 gm) or chicken (70 gm) or fish (100 gm).
✓ 2 chapattis (20 gm).
✓ Blended vegetables (100 gm).
✓ Curd (120 gm) or buttermilk.
✓ Plate of mixed greens (125 gm).

Sleep time:

✓ 200 ml milk.

UNMEASURED DIABETIC DIET:

Patients who are somewhat corpulent or of ordinary weight or the individuals who can't gauge their eating regimen, the unmeasured eating regimen is utilized. It alludes to the rundown of nourishment things which are classified into three in particular

✓ Food things to be stayed away from inside and out
✓ Food things to be taken in moderate sums
✓ Food things to be taken as wanted

Nourishment things to be maintained a strategic distance from out and out:

✓ Butter, Ghee
✓ Cakes and baked goods

- ✓ Condensed milk
- ✓ Cream and Cream Cheese
- ✓ Fried nourishment like bajji, vada and samosas
- ✓ Honey
- ✓ Ice cream, Kulfi and sweet
- ✓ Jam and Jelly
- ✓ Lemonade and other improved soda pops (circulated air through beverages)
- ✓ Marmalade
- ✓ Pies and puddings
- ✓ Sauces
- ✓ Sugar/Glucose, Jaggery
- ✓ Sweets, Chocolates
- ✓ Sweet bread rolls
- ✓ Sweetened pastries
- ✓ Tinned foods grown from the ground juices
- ✓ Wines and brew

Nourishment things to be taken in moderate sums:

- ✓ All sorts of bread
- ✓ Breakfast grains
- ✓ Diabetic nourishments
- ✓ Fresh products of the soil
- ✓ Macaroni, custard and nourishments with much flour
- ✓ Milk (full cream)
- ✓ Peas and heated beans
- ✓ Polished white rice
- ✓ Potatoes, sweet potatoes, colocasia and yam
- ✓ Rolls and crispbreads
- ✓ Wheat or bajra arrangements, suji, maida, sago and arrowroot

Nourishment things to be taken as wanted:

- ✓ All vegetables particularly green verdant vegetables (severe gourd, brinjal, cabbage, cauliflower, cucumber, drumsticks, ladyfinger, soybeans)

- ✓ Cheese
- ✓ Less sweet organic products like apple, guava, Jamun, orange, papaya
- ✓ Meat. Fish, eggs that are not singed
- ✓ Saccharine arrangements
- ✓ Skimmed milk
- ✓ Spices, salt, pepper and mustard
- ✓ Tea or espresso (without sugar)
- ✓ Tomato juice or lemon juice
- ✓ Wheat flour with wheat, darker rice, rice without starch water.

Focuses to be recollected:

- ✓ Eating while at the same time staring at the TV offers ascend to an admission of expanded calories.
- ✓ Eating when one is genuinely included (upbeat/dismal/irate/desolate) can offer ascent to over-eating or under-eating.
- ✓ Patients with high BP (Blood Pressure) ought to limit their salt admission.
- ✓ Special modifications in the eating routine ought to be put forth in defense of treatment with insulin infusions, diseases, regurgitating, social or strict get-togethers, fastings, and so forth.,
- ✓ Special care must be kept up on an eating routine while eating outside during shopping or on visit.
- ✓ Sugar-covered meds, biting gum, sodas, hack syrup and tonics ought to be utilized with alert.
- ✓ In this manner the eating regimen can be balanced relying upon the calories admission necessities as follows:
- ✓ By expanding the heaviness of wheat flour or bread cuts.
- ✓ By expanding the utilization of oil or ghee.
- ✓ By the expansion of spread.
- ✓ By changing skimmed milk to standard milk.

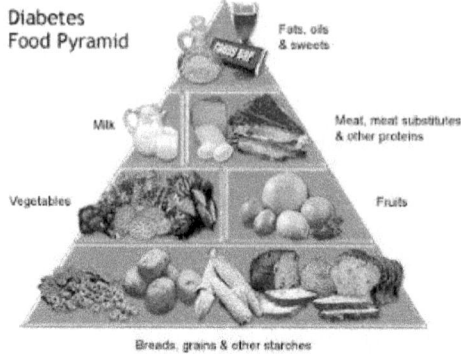

Diabetes Food Pyramid

Fats, oils & sweets

Milk

Meat, meat substitutes & other proteins

Vegetables

Fruits

Breads, grains & other starches

A HEALTHY PLATE YOU EAT TODAY, SO TOMORROW YOU CAN KEEP DISEASES AWAY

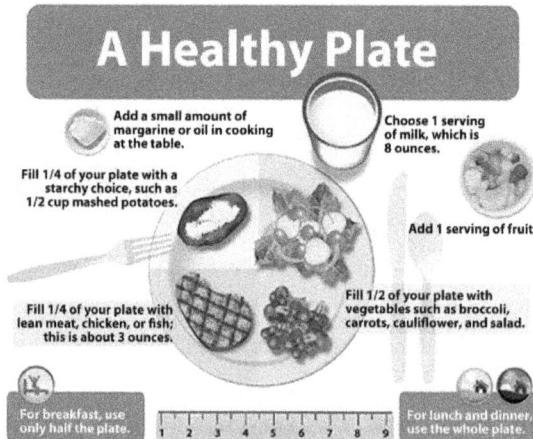

A Healthy Plate

Add a small amount of margarine or oil in cooking at the table.

Choose 1 serving of milk, which is 8 ounces.

Fill 1/4 of your plate with a starchy choice, such as 1/2 cup mashed potatoes.

Add 1 serving of fruit.

Fill 1/4 of your plate with lean meat, chicken, or fish; this is about 3 ounces.

Fill 1/2 of your plate with vegetables such as broccoli, carrots, cauliflower, and salad.

For breakfast, use only half the plate.

For lunch and dinner, use the whole plate.

Successful administration of diabetes can be accomplished with a fitting eating regimen. A portion of the diabetic weight control plans are depicted beneath:

(1)   GLYCEMIC INDEX (GI) DIET:

The glycemic record (GI) positions nourishment relying upon the rate at which the body separates it to frame glucose.

Low and High GI Foods:

110

The nourishments that are separated all the more gradually by the body are alluded to as Low GI nourishments. Instances of low GI nourishments incorporate entire grain bread, milk, beans, verdant vegetables and berries.

The nourishments that are immediately separated into glucose by the body are alluded to as High GI nourishments. Instances of High GI nourishments incorporate white bread, improved beverages, scones, potatoes and oranges.

Low GI nourishments don't cause a quick increment in glucose levels when contrasted with high GI nourishments and along these lines they are a superior alternative for keeping stable blood glucose levels. Low GI nourishments cause a person to feel increasingly fulfilled over a more drawn out period and less inclined to feel hungry before the following supper.

High GI nourishments can drive the body to create more insulin to balance with the brisk acting sugars and cause the person to feel hunger inside 2 to 3 hours, which can leave the calorie counter to pine for more nourishment. So individuals with diabetes should be cautious while taking high GI nourishment types.

Low GI foods grown from the ground:

- ✓ Berries, Grapes, Kiwi and Plums.
- ✓ Broccoli, Cabbage, Cauliflower, Lettuce and Peppers.

High GI foods grown from the ground:

- ✓ Bananas, Dates, Grapes, Mango, Oranges, Pears and Raisins.
- ✓ Beetroots, Carrots, Potatoes and Sweet corn.

Advantages of Low GI diets:

- ✓ Provide a drawn out arrival of vitality.
- ✓ Higher dietary benefit than high GI nourishments.
- ✓ Immediate interest for insulin is diminished after eating.

(2) GLYCEMIC LOAD:

Glycemic load is a grouping of various starches that estimates their effect on the body and glucose. It is determined by the accompanying equation:

GL = GI * Carbohydrate/100

One unit of GL approximates the impact of devouring 1 gram of glucose.

For instance, 1 cup of white rice serving size is 186 grams. Their GI is 64 and the all out starch is 52. At that point Glycemic Load (GL) is 33.28

GL = 64 * 52/100

GL = 33.28

The University of Sydney characterizes low, medium and high GL as follows:

- ✓ Low GL - 0 to 10
- ✓ Medium GL - 11 to19
- ✓ High GL - 20 and over

(3) LOW CARBOHYDRATE DIET:

Nourishments that contain effectively edible starches, for example, sugar, bread, pasta are constrained or supplanted with the nourishments containing a higher level of fats and moderate proteins (e.g., meat, fish, eggs) and different nourishments low in sugars (e.g., spinach serving of mixed greens vegetables).

These eating regimens are utilized to treat or forestall some constant illnesses and conditions like cardiovascular sicknesses, hypertension and diabetes.

- ✓ Moderate sugar - 130 to 225 gram of starches
- ✓ Low sugar - under 130 gram of starches
- ✓ Very low sugar - under 30 gram of starches

(4) LOW CARBOHYDRATE HIGH FAT (LCHF) DIET:

As the name proposes, the nourishments with high fat and low sugar are named as LCHF diet. This eating regimen is appropriate for individuals with type 2 diabetes and accommodating for the individuals who need to get in shape or keep up a solid weight.

Vegetables: Carrots, Cauliflower, Broccoli, Spinach.

Natural products: Apples, Blueberries, Oranges, Pears, Strawberries

Eggs: Omega-3 improved or fed eggs

Meat: Beef, Chicken, Lamb, Pork

(5) LOW-CALORIE DIET (LCD):

It is otherwise called Calorie confined eating routine. It is regularly prompted for individuals with diabetes who endeavor to accomplish weight reduction. National Health Service (NHS), England characterizes a low-calorie diet (kcal) of

- ✓ 1500 to 2000 calories/day for men
- ✓ 1000 to 1500 calories/day for ladies

1 kilocalorie (1 kcal) = 4.184 kilojoules (4 kJ)

Exceptionally Low-Calorie Diet (VLCD) is characterized as an eating routine with very or incredibly low day by day nourishment vitality utilization. They contain the prescribed day by day necessities for nutrients, minerals, follow components, unsaturated fats and proteins.

(6) LOW-FAT DIET:

A low-fat eating regimen is the one where the measure of fat we eat is confined. Low-fat eating regimen nourishments will in general diminish by and large calorie consumption and to improve cholesterol levels. Low-fat eating routine incorporates nourishments, for example, lentils, vegetables (carrots, broccoli, crude onion, garlic, lettuce), organic products (crude apples with skin, crude bananas, crude grapefruit), white fish, low-fat yogurt and cheddar, skinless chicken and turkey, entire grain food sources, for example, oats and high fiber bread.

(7) KETOGENIC DIET:

These eating regimens allude to any low sugar diet that consistently actuates ketosis. They are regularly higher in fat, lower in sugars and include satisfactory protein. These weight control plans are utilized to control epilepsy among youngsters. Those on ketogenic diets can encounter migraines, shortcoming, a sleeping disorder, blockage. Symptoms may likewise remember high centralizations of calcium for pee, kidney stones and sporadic periods.

(8) JUICING DIET:

It is a decent method for getting a solid measure of vegetables and organic products into one's eating regimen. A decent eating routine is the 80/20 guideline which prescribes

80% of juice from vegetables and 20% from natural products. These weight control plans help to lessen cerebrum mist, diminish exhaustion and improve by and large physical and emotional well-being.

Note: It is constantly fundamental to counsel your PCP first in the event that you are on diabetes prescription that can make hypoglycemic conditions happen.

13.DIABETES FOOD GROUPS

Individuals with diabetes need to comprehend which nourishments comprise of what, so blood glucose levels can be all around oversaw. The following are the nutrition types which ought to be taken by the diabetic individuals to deal with their eating routine simpler. Nourishment is partitioned into five primary gatherings as follows:

- ✓ Desserts and desserts
- ✓ Fruits
- ✓ High protein nourishments
- ✓ Non-bland vegetables
- ✓ Starchy nourishments

DESSERTS AND SWEETS:

They are not all that great for blood glucose levels. They ought to be taken in littler amounts or less frequently. Sugars can be utilized rather than sugars. Organic products, for example, berries can be utilized in making pastries and cake plans.

FRUITS:

Organic products are wealthy in supplements and fiber. They are likewise wealthy in fructose which raises glucose levels rapidly. So individuals with diabetes should take the one which doesn't raise glucose levels. For instance, Avocado (Persea Americana), Fig (Ficus carica), Guava (Psidium guajava) and Papaya (Carica papaya) can be taken by diabetic individuals.

- ✓ Avocados are pressed with carotenoids, help to get thinner, balance out glucose, brings down the danger of heart and heart infections and brings down cholesterol.
- ✓ Similarly, Figs assists with bringing down hypertension, get thinner, ensure against postmenopausal bosom disease, secure against macular degeneration and cardiovascular impacts.
- ✓ Guava is said to be diabetes-accommodating (because of rich fiber substance and low glycemic file), heart-accommodating (improve sodium and potassium parity of the body, brings down triglycerides and terrible cholesterol 'LDL', improves great cholesterol 'HDL'), brings down the danger of malignant growth, supports the safe framework, improves vision, treats blockage, ensures tooth and gums (because of intense calming and antibacterial capacity), help to get in shape, improves appearance and surface.
- ✓ Papaya contains an assortment of phytochemicals including carotenoids, polyphenols. They are additionally plentiful in fiber, Vitamin A, Vitamin C, flavonoids like beta-

115

carotene. They have cancer prevention agent movement. It supports up invulnerability, brings down cholesterol, helps weight reduction and decreases pressure, ensures against joint inflammation and malignancy, improves processing and visual perception, advances hair development and as an absolute sound organic product for diabetes.

HIGH PROTEIN FOODS:

MEAT:

Lean meat is a decent wellspring of protein with lower fat substance and in this way it is the lower calorie content. They help in building and fixing the body tissue. Protein can likewise be transformed into glucose if the body requires more vitality. Skinless chicken and fat cut off pork cleaves are instances of lean meat.

Red meat is a decent wellspring of protein and Vitamin B. They have a key job in the impact of the human eating routine. They have been connected with a few heart issues including type 2 diabetes and colorectal malignancy. These meat are gotten from ranch raised well evolved creatures, for example, pork, sheep, hamburger. They are additionally a rich wellspring of immersed fat, iron and zinc. Iron is expected to assist red with blooding cells transport oxygen. Zinc is required for DNA amalgamation and causes the resistant framework to work viably. Nutrient B6 and B12 are gainful for the safe framework and sensory system individually.

FISH:

It is a decent wellspring of protein. It contains omega 3, a basic unsaturated fat that enables dormant cerebrum to work. National Health Service prescribes an admission of two parts of fish for every week, wherein one bit must be of sleek fish.

EGGS, BEANS AND PULSES:

Eggs, beans and heartbeats have high proteins. Peas, chickpeas, runner   beans   and soya beans are remembered for this gathering. Eggs contain choline which is significant for cell films, mind and sensory system. Beans and heartbeats contain press and furnish fibre to help with assimilation.

DAIRY:

Dairy items are gotten from the creature's milk. They incorporate milk, cream, cheddar, spread and yogurt. Dairy nourishments contain a decent wellspring of calcium, protein and Vitamin B12. They contain a critical amount of fat which can expand the calories. Be that as it may, the low-fat dairy items are accessible for the individuals who wish to lessen the fat and calorie content from their day by day consumption.

The National Osteoporosis Society suggests an everyday admission of 700mg of calcium for grown-ups.

Lactose narrow mindedness:

It is generally normal and progressively predominant in Asian and African nations. Indications of lactose narrow mindedness incorporate stomach torments, feeling enlarged or encountering fart or loose bowels subsequent to having dairy items.

Full-fat dairy items have fatty substance and low-fat dairy items produced using skimmed milk offer a low-calorie elective.

NON STARCHY VEGETABLES:

These vegetables have low sugar content per 100 grams. Vegetables with 5 grams or less of sugars per 100 grams of weight are characterized as non-bland vegetables.

They are low in sugars and calories however wealthy in fiber and numerous supplements. They should make up half of our plate's substance at the primary suppers.

STARCHY FOODS:

They incorporate bland vegetables and entire grain nourishments. A fourth of the principle meals should be comprised of bland nourishments. Boring vegetables will be vegetables with a decent wellspring of fiber and different supplements. They have high sugar content. Entire grain foods are the boring nourishments produced using grains, for instance, grain, darker rice, wheat, oats and maize.

14.DIABETES DRINKS

The fundamental thought ought to be whether, or how much, the beverage will influence an individual glucose levels.

WATER:

It gives the hydration required by our body. Furthermore, is, obviously, zero sugar and zero calories. It is the perfect beverage for people with diabetes.

Diabetic individuals require increasingly liquid when blood glucose levels are high.

Having high blood glucose levels can expand the danger of drying out. Drinking water serves to rehydrate the blood when the body attempts to expel abundance glucose through pee. In the event that water get to is constrained, glucose may not be dropped of the pee, prompting further lack of hydration. Studies have additionally demonstrated that drinking water could assist control with blooding glucose levels.

The water admission by and large every day for men ought to be 2 liters (around ten 200ml glasses for each day) and ladies ought to be 1.6 liters (around eight 200ml glasses for each day). These liquid admission esteems can be comprised of any liquid despite the fact that water is the most strongly suggested.

MILK:

It has moderate sugar content that ought to be represented especially in type 1 diabetic individuals if drinking near or more than 100ml. Skimmed milk will in general have around a large portion of the calories of entire milk.

The quantity of calories down the middle a 16 ounces of milk differs from around 90 calories for skimmed milk to 190 calories for entire milk. [Note: half quart implies a unit of fluid or dry limit equivalent to one-eighth of a gallon. In Britain, it is equivalent to 0.568 liters and in the US, it is equivalent to 0.473 liters (for fluid measure) or 0.551 liters (for dry measure)]. Type 1 diabetic individuals need to deal with the starch substance of the milk when they are having a glass of it.

Milk contains lactose, a type of sugar which is separated into glucose in the small digestive tract. Individuals who are lactose narrow minded can separate the lactose gradually. This lactose goes through the stomach related framework and gets aged by gut microscopic organisms which prompts swelling, tooting and looseness of the bowels.

Individuals with lactose narrow mindedness need to maintain a strategic distance from or limit the admission of nourishments containing lactose, basically dairy nourishments, to forestall the above said side effects. In the event that an individual has a higher level of lactose bigotry, at that point he needs to maintain a strategic distance from or limit nourishments with littler measures of lactose including soups, bread and plate of mixed greens dressings.

COFFEE:

Moderate espresso utilization (2-3 cups every day) has given some medical advantages, including a lower danger of type 2 diabetes while high espresso utilization (at least 5 cups per day) has been connected with a higher hazard. Smooth espressos as lattes can be high in calories (100 to 300 calories).

Espresso has additionally been appeared to bring down dangers of the accompanying conditions as Endometrial malignant growth, forceful prostate disease, cardiovascular malady, strokes, Alzheimer's illness and Parkinson's sickness.

Espresso contains polyphenols that have cancer prevention agent and hostile to cancer-causing properties and assists with forestalling incendiary sicknesses. Espresso likewise contains the mineral magnesium and chromium. More noteworthy magnesium consumption has been connected with lower paces of type 2 diabetes.

TEA:

It is one of the solid beverage. Impact of non-smooth tea has a wide scope of medical advantages which remembers enhancements for insulin affectability, helps in keeping up sound circulatory strain, forestalling blood clusters, decreasing the danger of cardiovascular malady, diminishing the danger of creating type 2 diabetes and lessening the danger of creating malignancy, Teas, for example, dark tea, green tea contain polyphenols which may expand insulin movement. Polyphenols are known to have hostile to oxidative properties that can assist a person with protecting against irritation and cancer-causing agents. In 2002, American researchers found that the expansion of milk in tea diminished the insulin-sharpening impacts of tea. In 2009, Dutch researchers found that drinking three cups of tea could decrease the danger of creating type 2 diabetes by 40%

FRUIT JUICE:

Natural product juices have generally high sugar content. The calorie substance of natural product juice is like that of skimmed milk. Organic product juice is normally viewed as a solid alternative when it is taken in a genuine and unsweetened structure.

Standard utilization of natural product juice has been connected with an expansion in type 2 diabetes hazard. Beside Vitamin C and Calcium, they contain high calories (250ml glass of unsweetened squeezed orange ordinarily contains around 100 calories though genuine orange contains just 60 calories), fructose (a type of sugar) and absence of filaments (juice contains just less fiber and profoundly handled juices may not contain any fiber while entire organic product contains more fiber).

Dissolvable fiber (a sort of sugar) helps in bringing down cholesterol levels and improving blood glucose control whenever taken in huge sums. The entire organic product, for example, apples, oranges, pears contains progressively dissolvable filaments however not when squeezed. An ongoing report found that there is a connection between organic product juice and longer telomeres. Telomeres are defensive DNA on the finish of cell chromosomes. Longer telomeres are frequently connected with longer cell life expectancy, while short telomeres have been connected to insulin opposition and diabetes.

The generally high Glycemic file and high sugar substance of natural product juice help in raising glucose levels, on account of hyperglycemia. So it is smarter to have an entire natural product rather than organic product juices.

SUGARY SOFT DRINKS:

These beverages are usually alluded to as "full fat" drinks and often connected with less fortunate wellbeing whenever expended routinely. They are high in the two sugars and calories. They don't contain dietary benefit. It raises the dangers of stoutness, coronary illness and type 2 diabetes. It ought to be kept away from to forestall the ascent in blood glucose levels however it very well may be valuable to help the hypoglycemic patient when there is a need to raise their blood glucose levels.

Utilization of sugary could add to expanded weight gain. They quickly increment glucose levels and this can prompt tiredness and expanded yearning even in individuals without diabetes.

There is no particular suggested sugar admission for individuals with diabetes, yet they need to constrain their sugar consumption extensively less.

FRUIT SQUASH:

Squash doesn't convey the healthful advantages of genuine natural product squeeze yet can be a lower starch and lower-calorie option in contrast to sugary sodas.

DIET SOFT DRINKS:

Counterfeit sugars and other fake specialists to give sweetness, flavor and shading are utilized to set up these eating regimen sodas. The sugars used to set up these beverages are low in calories. Individuals ought to want to constrain or maintain a strategic distance from their introduction to these soda pops as a safety measure.

ALCOHOL:

Individuals with diabetes should be extra cautious with liquor. Distinctive mixed beverages will effectsly affect your glucose. It additionally relies upon the amount you drink. Liquor consumption fundamentally builds the danger of hypoglycemia (low glucose levels). Liquor restrains the liver from transforming proteins into glucose which implies you are at a more serious danger of hypoglycemia once your blood sugars begin to descend. A tremendous measure of liquor consumption prompts an ascent in glucose followed by a relentless drop a few hours after the fact, regularly during rest. Individuals who take insulin ought to be cautious about hypoglycemia. Observing blood glucose levels intently is a fundamental piece of dealing with your diabetes right now. On the off chance that your diabetes is as of now well leveled out, a moderate measure of liquor might be fine either previously, during or not long after a feast.

Drinking bunches of liquor can cause an expansion in pulse. These alcohols contain high calories which will prompt weight gain and neuropathic conditions by expanding agony and deadness.

Abstain from drinking on a vacant stomach, as this will rapidly build the measure of liquor in your circulation system. The suggested rules are two units for ladies and three units for men. In any case, it merits monitoring what number of units a beverage contains.

Generally speaking it is ideal to stay away from liquor drinking by diabetic individuals to have a solid existence.

ALCOHOL SUBSTITUTES:

Many substances can be used as alternatives to alcohol while cooking to tenderize meat. The alternative flavors to common alcohols (Beer, Brandy, Champagne, Red Burgundy, Red Wine, Rum, Sherry, White Burgundy, White Wine) for diabetic patients are Apple cider, Apricot syrup, Beef broth, Cherry cider syrup, Chicken broth, Diluted Cider Vinegar, Ginger ale, Orange juice, Peach syrup, Pear juice, Pineapple juice, Raspberry syrups, Red wine Vinegar, Spearmint extract, White grape juice.

15. DIABETES SWEETENERS

Sweeteners are of two types. They are Nutritive and Non-nutritive sweeteners.

NUTRITIVE SWEETENERS:

Nutritive sweeteners are those which have calories and provide nourishment. Examples are sugars and sugar alcohols.

(1) SUGARS:

Sugars are considered fine when they are eaten in moderation with a mixed meal and as part of a healthy overall diet. They do not cause special problems for people with carbohydrate intolerance such as diabetes mellitus or insulin resistance.

High intake of the substance can contribute to several health problems such as tooth decay, weight gain, obesity-related complications like type 2 diabetes, hypertension and heart disease. Problems such as osteoporosis and vitamin and mineral deficiencies can also occur when high-sugar foods replace more nutritionally balanced ones.

The major sources include sweets, chocolates, cakes and fruit drinks. The common sources of sugar on food and drinks include brown sugar, corn syrup, corn sweetener, dextrose, fructose, glucose, honey, lactose, maltose, sucrose, molasses, raw sugar and invert sugar. Some of them described below.

All sugars have 4 grams of carbohydrate per level teaspoon and 4 calories per gram.

- ✓ **SUCROSE**: It is a carbohydrate found in table sugar, cane sugar, raw sugar, brown sugar and powdered sugar. It is the primary sugar found in molasses and composed of 50% glucose and 50% fructose.
- ✓ **FRUCTOSE**: It is fruit sugar. It is a type of sugar found in plants. It is sweeter than sucrose. It is therefore used less as a sweetener.
- ✓ **DEXTROSE**: The D-isomer of glucose (D-glucose) is dextrose, occurs widely in nature.
- ✓ **CORN SUGAR**: This is also known as Corn syrup. This type of sugar is derived from corn starch and is high in glucose.
- ✓ **MALTOSE**: It is a potent sugar found in malt, beer and ales (brewed beer).
- ✓ **HFCS** (High Fructose Corn Syrup): It is sweeter than sucrose. It is a mixture of glucose and fructose that is usually added to sodas and soft drinks.
- ✓ **HONEY**: It is composed of 35% glucose and 40% fructose.

(1) SUGAR ALCOHOLS:

They are a type of carbohydrate called "polyols" which are used as alternative food sweeteners to natural sugars. They can contribute to weight gain if eaten in large enough quantities. They are also known for his or her potent laxative effect when eaten in excess.

- ✓ **SORBITOL**: It is a polyol derived from glucose. It is first discovered in 1872. It contains 60% of the sweetness of sucrose. Now it is commercially produced by the hydrogenation of glucose and is available in both liquid and crystalline form. It is useful in the production of confectionery, baked goods and chocolate where products tend to become dry or harden. It is non-cariogenic. It isn't utilized by oral microscopic organisms which separate sugars and starches to discharge acids that may prompt depressions or the disintegration of tooth polish. Sorbitol is slowly absorbed by the body, allowing a part of the ingested substance to succeed in the massive intestine where metabolism generates fewer calories.

- ✓ **XYLITOL**: It is derived from xylose. It is a white odorless crystalline powder that has been used as a sweetening agent in food. It is 100% as sweet as sucrose. It helps to prevent the development of dental caries (tooth decay). Products sweetened with xylitol creates an increase in salivary flow that helps repair damaged tooth enamel.

- ✓ **MANNITOL**: It is a polyol derived from mannose, Mannitol is about 70% as sweet as sucrose. It is non-cariogenic. It helps to prevent the development of dental caries (tooth decay). It is partially absorbed from the small intestine i.e., the ingested substance reaches the large intestine where metabolism yields fewer calories.

- ✓ **ISOMALT**: This is a sugar alcohol derived from sucrose and is around 60% as sweet as sucrose.

- ✓ **Hydrogenated Starch Hydrolysates** (HSH): It is derived from corn, wheat or potato starches. These sweeteners be present connecting 40% and 90% as sweet as sucrose.

NON - NUTRITIVE SWEETENERS:

These are counterfeit sugars. Low-calorie sugars are sugar substitutes that have zero calories and don't raise blood glucose levels which is an ideal decision for diabetic individuals over sugar. They are neither sugar nor fat. They give a critical improving impact without including starches or calories. They can be added to a diabetic dinner plan rather than traded.

(1)   SACCHARIN:

It was first found in 1878 by specialist Constantin Fahlberg. It is a counterfeit, non-nutritive sugar utilized in the creation of different nourishments and pharmaceutical items. It is regularly utilized in both hot and cold nourishments. It is 200 to multiple times better than sucrose (table sugar), doesn't raise glucose levels. Saccharin is temperamental when warmed yet doesn't respond artificially with other nourishment fixings, which makes it useful for capacity. It is regularly mixed with other fake sugars to make up for every sugar's shortcomings. Its utilization ought to be restricted in newborn children, youngsters and pregnant ladies. This is because of the plausibility of hypersensitive responses. They have a place with a class of mixes known as sulfonamides, which can cause hypersensitive responses in certain people. Responses can incorporate migraines, the runs, breathing challenges and skin issues.

(2)   ACESULFAME – K:

Acesulfame Potassium is a low-calorie sugar. It is multiple times as sweet as sucrose. It very well may be utilized in cooking on account of its capacity to oppose heat. It is generally added to dry blends for sans sugar gelatins, sweets and drinks, and can likewise be utilized in heated products.

(3)   ASPARTAME:

It was first found in 1965 by a scientist called James M. Schlatter. It is a counterfeit, non-nutritive sugar that is multiple times better than sucrose (table sugar). It has been utilized as a tabletop sugar since 1970. It isn't steady in heat or for significant stretches in fluid structure and is along these lines not utilized in cooking. It is additionally regularly remembered for pharmaceutical medications and enhancements. The adequate every day consumption (ADI) of 40 mg/kg of body weight of aspartame was altogether sheltered aside from individuals with the hereditary condition phenylketonuria (PKU).

Advantages:

- ✓ Only a minor measure of aspartame is expected to create a sweet taste, which implies that its caloric commitment is immaterial.
- ✓ The sweetness of aspartame endures longer sucrose.
- ✓ They contain zero sugars and accordingly doesn't affect blood glucose levels.
- ✓ Impediments:
- ✓ It has been connected with the improvement or disturbance of a few wellbeing conditions, for example, diabetes mellitus, seizures, cerebral pains, melancholy, mental states, hyperthyroidism, hypertension, joint inflammation.
- ✓ It has likewise been connected with the improvement of cerebrum disease in warm blooded creatures, for example, rodents and monkeys.

(4)   SUCRALOSE:

It was found in 1976 by researchers from Tate and Lyle, working with specialists Leslie Hough and Shashikant Phadnis at Queen Elizabeth College, London. Sucralose is around 320 to multiple times better than sucrose, twice as sweet as saccharin, and multiple times as sweet as aspartame. It is steady under warmth and over an expansive scope of pH conditions. Subsequently, it tends to be utilized in preparing or in items that require a more drawn out time span of usability. Research shows it has no impact on glucose and is considered safe for use in all age populaces, including pregnant ladies and youngsters.

(5) CYCLAMATE:

It was found at the University of Illinois in 1937. It is the conventional term for the cyclohexylsulfamates. It is a without calorie sugar that is multiple times better than sucrose. It is dissolvable in fluids and on the grounds that it is steady in warmth and cold, it has a long timeframe of realistic usability. It is presently prohibited in many nations because of its connection with expanded malignant growth chance.

PHYSICAL EXERCISE:

Exercise is a significant piece of the treatment program both for Type 1 (who are underweight) and Type 2 Diabetes (who are overweight) patients. An individual is viewed as overweight or fat dependent on his Body Mass Index which is determined as follows:

Weight Index (BMI) = Weight (kg)/Height (m2)

Men are viewed as stout or overweight if their BMI is more than 30 and ladies if their BMI is more than 28.6.

Benefits of exercise:

(1) Weight Reduction:

This is particularly significant for patients with type 2 diabetes who are hefty. Diabetes is restored and controlled after they have lost adequate load to accomplish the ideal weight. The system of this change is the expansion in the quantity of insulin receptors on getting in shape. This expansion is exceptionally successful in controlling diabetes.

(2) Increased efficacy of insulin:

In patients with type 1 diabetes where there is a finished lack of insulin, practice lessens the necessity of insulin by expanding the affectability of the body to insulin. In type 2 diabetes where next to no insulin is accessible in the pancreas, exercise can expand the viability of whatever insulin is accessible in the body. At the point when fat people get more fit, the quantity of insulin receptors increments and thus and every cell gets its ordinary portion of glucose and furthermore the blood level of glucose standardizes. In this manner getting in shape intends to control or even fix diabetes.

(3) Reduced risk for heart disease:

Fat gets stored in the veins that diminishes the blood dissemination and offer ascent to respiratory failures. Exercise expands the effectiveness of the heart to siphon blood just as by expanding levels of High-thickness Lipoprotein (HDL's) in the blood. These HDL's abatement the fat substance in blood and improve blood course.

(4) Blood Pressure Normalization:

High BP is related with diabetes. Exercise improves the flow of blood in the heart and kidneys in this manner forestalling the affidavit of fat in the veins that lead to normalizing circulatory strain.

(5) Relieves stress and strain:

Exercise diminishes physical and mental pressures, stress and strains. Normal exercise causes the patient to feel dynamic, good and merry.

Benefits Of Moderate Exercise And Diabetes

- **Benefits Of Exercise**
  - 1) Weight Loss
  - 2) Lower Blood Pressure
  - 3) Reduce Risk for Heart Disease
  - 4) Improve Cholesterol Ratios
  - 5) Control Blood Sugar
  - 6) Reduce Back and Joint Pain
  - 7) Improve Balance
  - 8) Reduce Medications
  - 9) Increase Self Confidence
  - 10) Reduce Risk For Fall

Types of exercise:

Every diabetic must be assessed by the doctor to settle on the kind of activity that must be embraced by him. Exercise can be evaluated into three as follows:

- ✓ Mild - Boating, Cycling, Gardening, Golf, Jogging, Walking.
- ✓ Moderate - Badminton, Bowling in cricket, Swimming, table tennis.
- ✓ Severe - Skin, Squash, Ice skating, Running, Tennis and Mountain Climbing.

Frequency of exercise:

Normal exercise can realize the molding of the heart. This forestalls coronary failures and keeps the individual new and fit for the duration of the day. Exercise during ailment, extraordinary climate conditions isn't fitting and if basic, a relative ought to go with the patient to forestall low glucose levels.

YOGA:

Yoga is an antiquated Indian system of incorporating human character at the physical, mental, good and profound levels. The act of yoga serves to co-ordinate the breath, brain and body to advance unwinding, create breath mindfulness and give a feeling of inward harmony. It includes different body stances and developments (known as asanas), breathing methods and reflection which are altogether intended to advance physical solace and mental self-restraint.

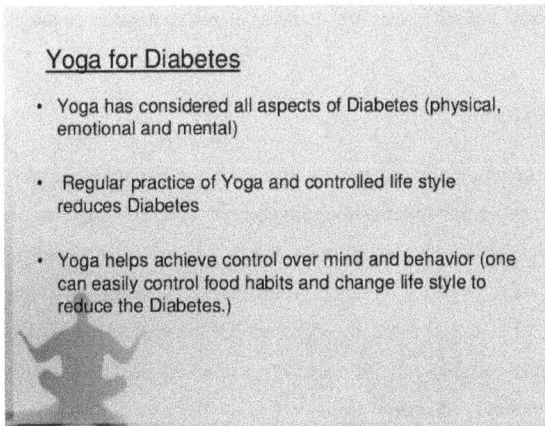

Yoga for Diabetes

- Yoga has considered all aspects of Diabetes (physical, emotional and mental)

- Regular practice of Yoga and controlled life style reduces Diabetes

- Yoga helps achieve control over mind and behavior (one can easily control food habits and change life style to reduce the Diabetes.)

Potential instruments:

- ✓ Glucagon discharge is upgraded by pressure. Yoga viably diminishes pressure, in this way lessening glucagon and perhaps improving insulin activity.
- ✓ Weight misfortune prompted by yoga is a well-acknowledged system.
- ✓ Muscular unwinding, advancement and improved blood supply to muscles may upgrade insulin receptor articulation on muscles causing expanded glucose take-up by muscles and consequently diminishing glucose.
- ✓ Blood pressure assumes an incredible job in the advancement of diabetic and related inconveniences, which is demonstrated to be profited by yoga. Similar holds for expanded cholesterol levels.
- ✓ Yoga decreases adrenaline, noradrenalin and cortisol in the blood, which is named as pressure hormones. This is a presumable system of progress in insulin activity.
- ✓ Many yogic stances do create stretch on the pancreas, which is probably going to animate the pancreatic capacity.
- ✓ Advantages of Yoga:
- ✓ Better rest.
- ✓ Reduced uneasiness and wretchedness.
- ✓ Enhanced sentiments of prosperity.
- ✓ Relief from constant diseases.
- ✓ Improved absorption, course, and insusceptibility.
- ✓ Improved stance, adaptability and quality.
- ✓ Enhanced fixation and vitality levels.
- ✓ Enhanced capacity and effectiveness of respiratory, neurological and endocrine organs.

Care - MEDITATION:

Care is a system embraced to getting mindful of minute by-minute contemplations, feelings and physical sensations in a non-judgemental way. The establishments of care lie in the antiquated act of contemplation; care can be received and rehearsed by anybody independent of social or strict direction. Care can assist break with bringing down the consistent pattern of getting focused, on edge and discouraged. Weights and strains of regular day to day existence cause an interior clash of evasion and fascination. Individuals endeavor to maintain a strategic distance from 'negative feelings', for example, blame, pity, disappointment and outrage and rather are pulled in to sentiments of bliss and satisfaction.

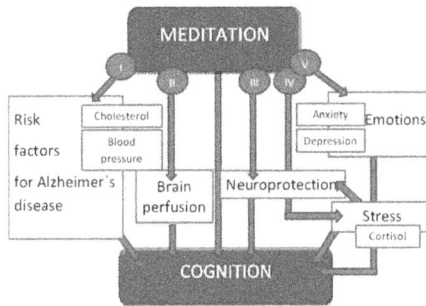

Care energizes consideration and spotlights on the present minute and the advancement of non-judgemental cognizance, this permits the individual to acknowledge the manner in which they are feeling as opposed to continually doing combating to attempt to transform it. Care based methodologies are especially viable in supporting diabetes the board and the psychological strife that is joined by a determination of, for example, constant physical disease. It can address the sentiments of blame, outrage and help self-acknowledgment to support the satisfaction of an unhindered life. Care has likewise been found to have an improved clinical impact of glycemic control so it helps mental wellbeing as well as might positively affect the administration of the physical condition.

16.ACUPRESSURE

Pressure point massage is innocuous restoring for Diabetes. Pressure point massage is an antiquated Chinese procedure mends Diabetes. Pressure point massage is useful in different infections like Headache, Migraine, Sinus Congestion, Eyestrain, Nasal Problems, Asthma, Anxiety, Diabetes, and so forth. Pressure point massage has different constrain focuses on body spots to fix Diabetes.

9 Best Acupressure points for Diabetes:

(1) Spleen point (Lower Leg Point):

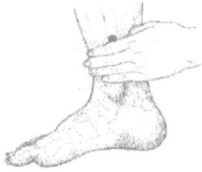

(2) Liver point (Foot Toe Point):

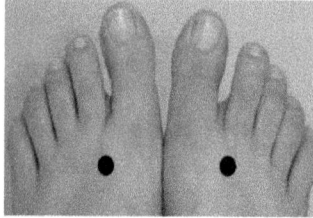

(3) Kidney point (Inner Foot Point):

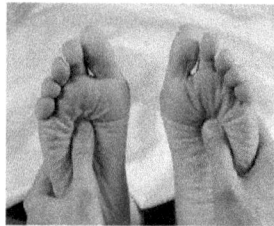

(4) Stomach point (Inner Low Leg Point):

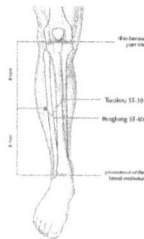

(5) Arthritis point:

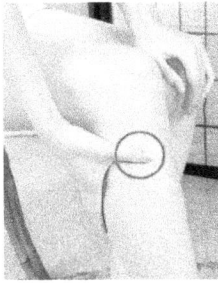

(6) Intestine point:

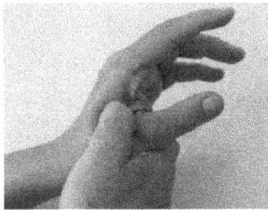

(7) Urinary point:

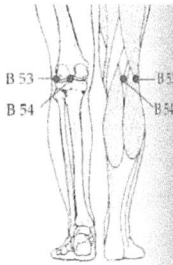

B 53   B 53
B 54   B 54

(8) Stress Relief point:

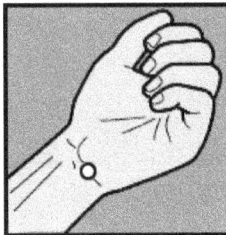

(9) Big Toe point:

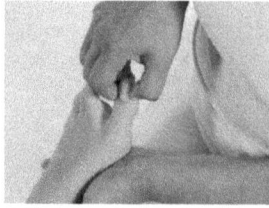

Effects of Acupressure:

✓ It decreases the torment of various sorts, for example, joint agony, cerebral pain, spinal pain, toothache and sprains.

✓ It has a sedating or narcotic impact on the cerebrum.

✓ It fortifies the body's characteristic opposition power because of which the respiratory rate, heartbeat, circulatory strain, temperature and digestion become typical.

✓ Depression, Anxiety, Stress and Tension are controlled with pressure point massage because of its impact on the mind.

✓ Points of interest of Acupressure:

✓ An simple, basic and successful type of treatment.

✓ No cash is required.

✓ No reactions.

✓ It should be possible by claim and however many occasions as could be expected under the circumstances.

✓ It builds the proficiency of organs and frameworks of the body.

✓ Even in genuine ailments, it forestalls the disturbance of indications.

✓ It gives a rapid help when it is trailed by different types of treatment.

Needle therapy:

Customary Chinese Medicine (TCM) is an old type of treatment that is bit by bit picking up acknowledgment in the western world. Right now needles are utilized to invigorate different focuses in the body. It effect sly affects the body like – pain relieving, calming, Homeostatic, Immune upgrading, and sedating impacts. It is all around utilized in the treatment of Paralysis, Migraine, Insomnia, Sciatica, Cerebral paralysis, spondylosis, Sinusitis, Spinal rope issue, and so forth.,

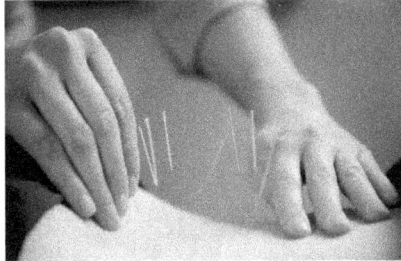

Effects in Diabetes:

- ✓ Lower blood glucose content.
- ✓ Lower the arrival of pancreatic glucagon.
- ✓ Attenuate indications of polyphagia (the desire to eat excessively), polydipsia (over the top thirst) and polyuria (inordinate section of pee).
- ✓ Prevent the easing back of engine nerve conduction.
- ✓ Improve microcirculation and myocardial contractility.
- ✓ Enhance blood surge and manage vascular fringe opposition.
- ✓ Exert antiatherogenic, cancer prevention agent and immunomodulating impacts.
- ✓ Obliterate antherosclerosis of the legs.
- ✓ Induce discharge of endogenous beta-endorphin.
- ✓ Elevate a brought down agony limit.
- ✓ Increase cell multiplication and neuropeptide Y levels.

BACK RUB THERAPY AND REFLEXOLOGY:

Back rub treatment could be fused into unwinding treatment, yet it likewise fills another need that can be especially valuable for individuals with diabetes. By capably working the body's tissue, back rub can animate better blood development around the body. Improved dissemination can do ponders for diabetic neuropathy and different diabetes-related intricacies. The back rub takes numerous structures, some of which might be more reasonable for diabetics than others.

Reflexology alludes to the type of treatment which includes offering back rub to certain reflex regions of the feet and hands.

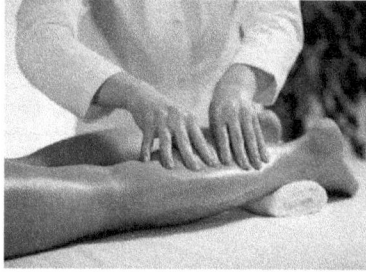

Fragrance based treatment:

Fragrance based treatment is the act of using fundamental oils (separated from plants and thought) to improve the state of the psyche or body. Oils may invigorate, unwind, steady, sterilize, against kindle, decongest and significantly more. They are conveyed to the body nasally through a vaporizer, a tissue or now and then by means of a shower or back rub. Utilized close by different medicines, fragrance based treatment can offer advantages to individuals with diabetes. There is a solid assemblage of proof that proposes fragrant healing can lessen diabetes-related pressure, and enhance some other enthusiastic issues. Fragrance based treatment can likewise be utilized to decrease the impacts of some diabetic inconveniences, explicitly those influencing the skin, for example, ulcers.

Diabetes and Blood Sugar

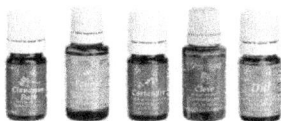

Mix equal parts Cinnamon Bark, Fennel, Coriander, Clove, and Dill in a capsule. Take 2 times daily.

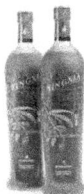

Apply 2 drops of Thieves and Lemongrass (along with any of the other oils above) and apply to the pancreas Vita Flex Points on the feet 2 times daily.

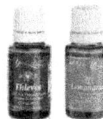

Drink 1 ounce of NingXia Red 3 times daily.

Take 2 drops of Ocotea under the tongue 2-3 times daily.

Adjust routine based on your blood sugar readings. Use in conjunction with a healthy diet and exercise.

MUSIC THERAPY:

Music treatment is a type of treatment utilizing music, instruments to reestablish, keep up and improve physical, physiological and profound wellbeing and prosperity.

General Benefits:

- ✓ It produces a decrease in nervousness and stress.
- ✓ It can acquire positive changes temperament and passionate states.
- ✓ It can reduce muscle pressure achieving unwinding of the body.
- ✓ This kind of treatment is delighted in by all.
- ✓ The length of remain in the emergency clinic or treatment period is diminished.
- ✓ An passionate bond creates between the patient, his relatives and specialists.
- ✓ Advantages in Diabetics:
- ✓ Increases the stomach related and metabolic action in the body. In this way expanding the emission of stomach related chemicals and hormones including insulin.
- ✓ Stabilizes the circulatory strain, pulse and subsequently forestalls confusions of the heart.
- ✓ Major factors in diabetes, for example, mental pressure and strain are controlled.
- ✓ The resistant framework gets helped up and battles different sicknesses in the body.

Ragas helpful for the treatment of Diabetes:

The accompanying ragas are helpful in the treatment of diabetes: Raga Kalingara, Raga Hindol, Raga Bhairav, Raga Kafi, Raga Hansdhwani, Raga Bahar, Raga Deshkar, Raga Lalit and Raga Jaijaiwanti.

BIOFEEDBACK:

Biofeedback, or applied psychophysiological input, is a patient-guided treatment that shows a person to control muscle pressure, torment, internal heat level, cerebrum waves, and other real capacities and procedures through unwinding, representation, and other subjective control strategies. The name biofeedback alludes to the organic signals that are bolstered back, or returned, to the patient for the patient to create procedures of controlling them.

Clinical biofeedback systems that became out of the early research center methodology are presently generally used to treat an ever-extending rundown of conditions. These incorporate headache cerebral pains, strain migraines and numerous different kinds of torment, High pulse, low circulatory strain, sporadic pulses and epilepsy.

The "Muscle Whistler", appeared here with surface EMG (Electromyogram) terminals, was an early biofeedback gadget created by Dr. Harry Garland and Dr. Roger Melen in 1971.

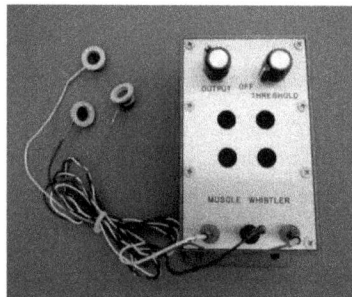

Biofeedback utilizes an extraordinarily structured machine that records muscle withdrawals and skin temperature utilizing sensors. Utilizing this machine, you can start to get familiar with the essential standards of controlling your body. Biofeedback could be especially valuable for individuals with diabetes who are additionally inclined to cerebral pains (as poor vision brought about by diabetic retinopathy can cause migraines).

17. AYURVEDIC HERBAL MEDICINE

Ayurveda began in Bharat long back in the pre-Vedic sum. Rigveda and Atharva-Veda (5000 years B.C.), the most punctual archived antiquated Indian information has references on wellbeing and sicknesses. Ayurveda writings like Charak Samhita and Sushruta Samhita were recorded concerning a thousand years B.C. The term Ayurveda signifies 'Study of Life'. It manages measures for stimulating living all through the total range of life and its various stages. In addition, adapting to standards for the upkeep of wellbeing, it has likewise built up a wide scope of helpful measures to battle sickness. Therefore Ayurveda gets probably the most established arrangement of social insurance managing both the preventive and remedial parts of life in a most complete manner and presents a nearby closeness to the WHO's idea of wellbeing propounded inside the time. An investigation of its numerous old style treatises shows the nearness of 2 schools of Physicians and Surgeons and eight strengths. These eight controls are for the most part called "Ashtanga Ayurveda" Herbs and an exacting eating routine make up the premise of the treatment. Yoga treatment is a piece of the Ayurvedic treatment framework and is regular all through the UK.

Ayurvedic herbs for Diabetes:

1. *Cassia auriculata*

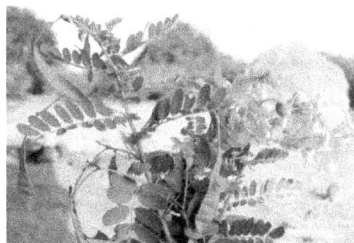

The roots are astringent, cooling, alterative, depurative and exoteric, and are valuable in skin maladies, uncleanliness, tumors,asthma and urethrorrhoea. The leaves are exchange, and a decoction of this is utilized as purifications and washes. The leaves are depurative and anthelmintic and are prescribed for uncleanliness, skin sicknesses and ulcers. The blossoms are utilized in diabetes, urethrorrhoea, nighttime emanations and pharyngopathy. The seeds are astringent. Harsh, cooling blocking, depurative, Spanish fly, anthelmintic, stomachic and exoteric, and are helpful in diabetes, chyluria, ophthalmia, looseness of the bowels, the runs, swellings, stomach issue, uncleanliness, skin sicknesses, worm invasions and constant purulent conjunctivitis.

2. *Vinca rosea.L*

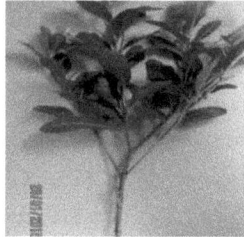

The natural product is a couple of follicles 2-4cm long and 3mm expansive. In Ayurveda for (Indian customs medication) the concentrate of its underlying foundations and shoots, however toxic, is utilized against a few sicknesses. In conventional Chinese medication, extricates from it have been utilized against various infections, including diabetes, intestinal sickness and hodkin's lymphoma.

3. Haridra (Curcuma longa) –

Commonly called turmeric. It is called as Manjal in Tamil. It is an enemy of malignant growth, calming, hostile to diabetic herb which treats different maladies including diabetes.

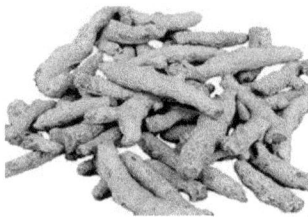

4. Lashun (Allium sativum) –

Garlic is another common solution for diabetes. It is called as Poondu in Tamil. It contains allicin, which helps in decreasing the sugar level in the blood. It additionally realizes the deterioration of cholesterol in the body.

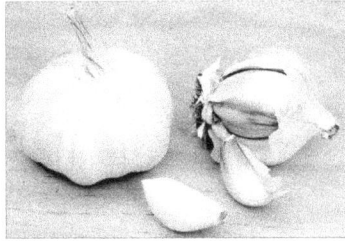

5. Jamun (Syzygium cumini) –

Commonly known as Jambul, Jambolan, Jamun and in Tamil, it is called Naval. It is an evergreen tree, whose seeds contain jamboline, which is valuable in patients with diabetes. Jamboline forestalls the change of starch into sugar and furthermore lessens sugar amount in pee and diminishes thirst.

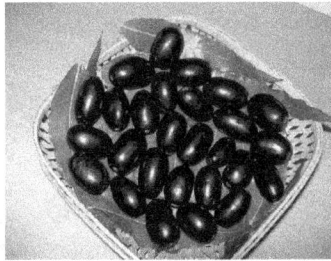

6. Karela (Momordica charantia) –

It is unpleasant melon, harsh gourd and in Tamil, it is known as Paagar kaai. It is a climber developed as a vegetable harvest. The organic product contains certain insulin-like mixes, which decrease blood glucose levels and furthermore helps in animating the arrival of insulin from the pancreas. It can likewise diminish raised blood cholesterol levels and furthermore forestall ketosis.

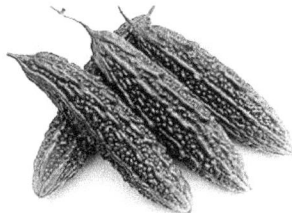

7. Neem (Azadirachta indica) –

Vembu in Tamil. It has germ-free properties and is helpful in mending diabetic foot, gangrene and goes about as a blood purifier and secures veins against infection.

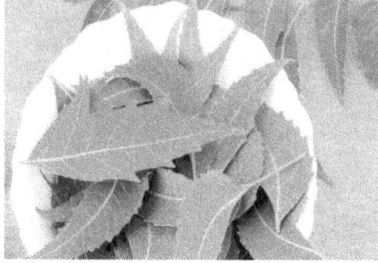

8. Sadabahar (Vinca rosea) –

Nithya Kalyani in Tamil. This blossom is found in numerous assortments and numerous hues like pink, white, and so on. Utilize the leaves of sadabahar for diabetes. Eat 2-3 blossoms in a vacant stomach and bubble water with blossoms and drink it. It is profoundly useful to fix diabetes. It is likewise known for its disease fix.

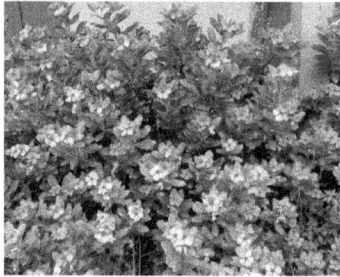

9. Abhraka Bhasma –

It is an Ayurvedic mineral-based drug, arranged from sanitized dark Mica. It is utilized in the treatment of asthma, heart infections, urinary issue, wretchedness, uneasiness, skin sicknesses, stress issue, and so on.

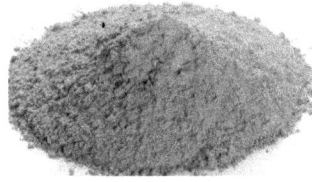

10.Aloe Vera

In fundamental human clinical examinations, the gel has indicated huge outcomes in the treatment of asthma, peptic ulcers, and diabetes mellitus. The gel has been sold in the wellbeing nourishment advertise as a tonic, just as for "supporting the resistant framework" and "supporting sound relaxing". Remotely, the gel has been utilized from numerous points of view: beauty care products, dermabrasion, wound-mending, and psoriasis. In beautifying agents, the gel is added to creams, chemicals, shampoos, suntan salves, and burn from the sun medications The medication got from aloe latex is a piece of one of the most grounded anthraquinone bunches that capacity as energizer diuretics. The latex is formally endorsed as a diuretic in the U.S., England, and Germany.

The German Commission E prescribes the utilization of aloe for infrequent obstruction and for conditions that require a delicate stool, for example, butt-centric crevices, hemorrhoids, and after rectal or butt-centric medical procedure. Remotely, the latex is utilized as the gel and as a calming specialist in treating consumes and gentle cuts.

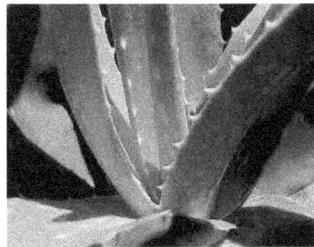

Benefits of using Ayurvedic medicines:

➢ Stimulates the discharge of insulin from the pancreas, which is the significant deformity in diabetes.

- It improves starch digestion and accordingly decrease the glucose levels in the blood.
- Enhance the fat digestion to diminish the degree of cholesterol, lipids and triglycerides which can likewise help in forestalling difficulties of heart and mind stroke and ketosis.
- Relief of side effects like expanded thirst, pee and tiredness, and so on.,
- Certain fixings forestall kidney intricacies (Albuminuria), Diabetic Retinopathy, Skin diseases and genitourinary frameworks.

Normal home solution for diabetes:

(1) Using severe gourd

- ✓ Remove the skin and seeds of 4 to 5 severe gourds.
- ✓ Crush them to make a glue.
- ✓ Press this glue on a sifter and concentrate the juice.
- ✓ Drink this juice on an unfilled stomach each morning.

(2) Using Cinnamon powder

- ✓ Boil 1 liter of water and let it be in stew for 20 minutes on low fire.
- ✓ While stewing, include 3 teaspoons of cinnamon powder.
- ✓ Strain the blend.
- ✓ Drink the whole measure of this water each day.

(3) Using Fenugreek seeds

- ✓ Take 4 tablespoons of fenugreek seeds and absorb them 250 ml of water medium-term.
- ✓ Crush them toward the beginning of the day and strain the blend and gather the water.
- ✓ Drink it consistently for 2 months.

18. HOMEOPATHY:

Homeopathy is a kind of treatment that is totally founded on the utilization of exceptionally weakened substances. In huge portions, these substances are hurtful however in little doses, they can be gainful to the body, making it recuperate itself. Homeopathy is one of a few integral of elective medications - for example medications that contrast from ordinary Western prescription - that are utilized to treat a wide scope of physical and mental conditions, including diabetes.

Fundamental standards of homeopathy:

Homeopathy is a powerful, non-obtrusive framework dependent on fixed laws and standards. Its logical way to deal with parts of the illness incorporates

- ✓ The law of comparative
- ✓ The Law of weakening (recuperating or little portion)
- ✓ The rule of potentisation

The fundamental idea of homeopathy is treating like with likes, utilizing cures that are fit for delivering in sound people comparative indications as those accomplished by the patient. By intensely weakening and shaking substances that cause certain indications, homeopathy professionals guarantee these equivalent substances can be utilized to evacuate those manifestations. They additionally accept that the more a substance is weakened, through a procedure known as succussion, the more prominent its capacity to treat side effects.

After the patient is inspected, the homeopath will endorse a treatment plan comprising of homeopathic treatments as a pill, case or tincture. Follow-up arrangements may likewise be prescribed to survey how viable the treatment is demonstrating.

19.ALLOPATHY

There are a wide range of sorts of hostile to diabetic medications which incorporate oral drugs, insulin infusions and insulin siphons.

(1) Oral Medications:

Type 2 diabetes results when the body can't create the measure of insulin it needs to change over nourishment into vitality or when it can't utilize insulin suitably. Now and then the body is delivering more insulin than is required by an individual to keep blood glucose in an ordinary range. However blood glucose stays high in light of the fact that the body's cells are impervious with the impacts of insulin. Doctors and researchers accept that type 2 diabetes is brought about by numerous components, including lacking insulin and insulin obstruction. They progressively accept that the relative commitment each factor makes toward causing diabetes differs from individual to individual.

(2) Insulin:

Insulin is a hormone made by the pancreas that allows your body to use sugar (glucose) from starches in the sustenance that you eat for essentialness or to store glucose for at some point later. Insulin helps keeps your glucose level from getting unreasonably high (hyperglycemia) or exorbitantly low (hypoglycemia).

The cells in your body need sugar for essentialness.In any case, sugar can't go into the greater part of your cells straightforwardly. After you eat nourishment and your glucose level ascents, cells in your pancreas (known as beta cells) are motioned to discharge insulin into your circulatory system. Insulin at that point appends to and signals cells to assimilate sugar from the circulatory system. Insulin is regularly portrayed as a "key," which opens the cell to permit sugar to enter the cell and be utilized for vitality.

Insulin, got from the Latin word "insula" which means island) is a peptide hormone delivered by beta cells of the pancreatic islets. The pancreatic beta cells (β cells) are known to be delicate to the glucose focus in the blood. At the point when the blood glucose levels are high they discharge insulin into the blood; when the levels are low they stop their emission of this hormone into the general dissemination.

You can infuse insulin into your stomach area, upper arm, bum, hip and the front or side of the thigh. Insulin works quickest when it is infused into the guts.

In the occurrence to contain supplementary sugar in your body than it requirements, insulin helps store the sugar in your liver and discharges it while your glucose level is low or on the off chance that you need more sugar, for example, in the middle of suppers or during physical action. In this manner, insulin assists offset with excursion glucose levels and keeps them in an ordinary range. As glucose levels increase, the pancreas secretes supplementary insulin.

In the event that your body doesn't deliver enough insulin or your cells are impervious with the impacts of insulin, you may create hyperglycemia (high glucose), which can cause long haul difficulties if the glucose levels remain raised for significant stretches.

Insulin Treatment for Diabetes

Individuals with type 1 diabetes can't make insulin in light of the fact that the beta cells in their pancreas are harmed or crushed. In this way, these individuals will require insulin infusions to permit their body to process glucose and evade confusions from hyperglycemia.

Individuals with type 2 diabetes don't react well or are impervious to insulin. They may require insulin shots to assist them with bettering procedure sugar and to forestall long haul intricacies from this illness. People through type 2 diabetes might originally exist treated with oral meds, alongside diet and exercise. Since type 2 diabetes is a dynamic condition, the more somebody has it, the almost certain it will expect insulin to keep up glucose levels.

Different sort of insulin be utilize to treat diabetes and comprise:

Quick acting insulin: It begins working around 15 minutes after infusion and tops at roughly 1 hour yet keeps on working for two to four hours. This is generally taken before a supper and notwithstanding long-acting insulin.

Short-acting insulin: It begins working roughly 30 minutes after infusion and tops at around 2 to 3 hours yet will keep on working for three to six hours. It is generally given before a dinner and notwithstanding long-acting insulin.

Middle acting insulin: It begins working roughly 2 to 4 hours after infusion and pinnacles around 4 to 12 hours after the fact and keeps on laboring for 12-18 hours. It is typically taken two times every day and notwithstanding a fast or short-acting insulin.

Long-acting insulin: It begins working following a few hours after infusion and works for roughly 24 hours. In the event that fundamental, it is frequently utilized in blend with fast or short-acting insulin.

Insulin can be given by a syringe, infusion pen, or an insulin siphon that conveys a constant progression of insulin.

Your primary care physician will work with you to make sense of which sort of insulin is best for you relying upon whether you have type 1 or type 2 diabetes, your glucose levels and your way of life.

At the point when the pancreatic beta cells are obliterated by an immune system process, insulin can never again be combined or be emitted into the blood. This outcomes in type 1 diabetes mellitus, which is portrayed by high glucose levels, and summed up body squandering, which is deadly if not treated. This must be amended by infusing the hormone, either straightforwardly into the blood if the patient is extremely sick and confounded or torpid, or subcutaneously for routine upkeep treatment, which must be proceeded for the remainder of the individual's life

In type 2 diabetes mellitus the pulverization of beta cells is less articulated than in type 1 diabetes, and presumably not because of an immune system process. Rather, there is a gathering of amyloid in the pancreatic islets, which upsets the life structures and physiology of the pancreatic islets.

It wasn't until 1921 that insulin was genuinely extricated. This was finished by a group from the University of Toronto which included Frederick Banting and J Macleod, who was given the Nobel Prize in Physiology or Medicine in 1923.

Insulin Pens

Insulin pens got their name since they are about the size and state of a composing pen. They contain insulin (rather than ink) and have a dial for setting the portion. A dispensable pen needle is connected as far as possible of the pen before infusing it. Just like the case with syringes, pen needles are accessible in an assortment of lengths and thicknesses. Since they cut down on restorative waste and are considered by most to be increasingly advantageous, precise and simple to use than syringes, insulin pens are developing in fame among individuals everything being equal.

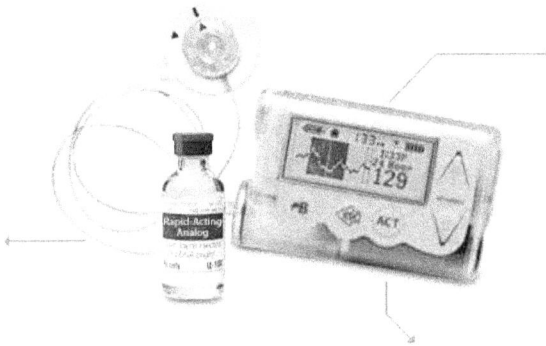

Check the pen:

Guarantee that it contains the best possible kind of insulin and contains enough to cover your full portion. Additionally, check to ensure that the lapse date has not passed.

Type	Brand Name	When to take	Onset
"Rapid-acting"	Novolog Humalog Apidra Afreeza	Inject/inhale immediately before or after eating	Starts working in 15 minutes
"Short-acting"	Humulin R Novolin R	Inject 30-60 minutes before eating	Starts working in 30-60 minutes
"Intermediate"	Humulin N Novolin N	Inject twice a day, in the morning and evening (typical use)	Starts working in 1-3 hours
"Long-Acting"	Lantus Levemir	Take at the same time everyday	Lasts 18-24 hours
"Pre-mixed"	Humalog Mix 75/25 Humalog Mix 50/50 Novolog Mix 70/30 Humulin 70/30 Humulin 50/50	Varies but typically twice daily	Varies

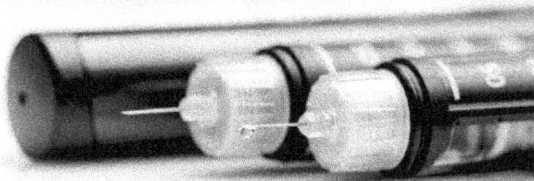

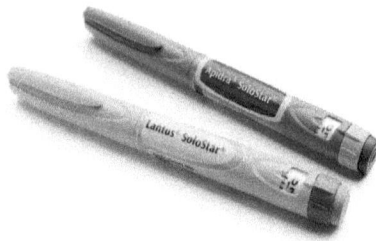

Innsulin Pen

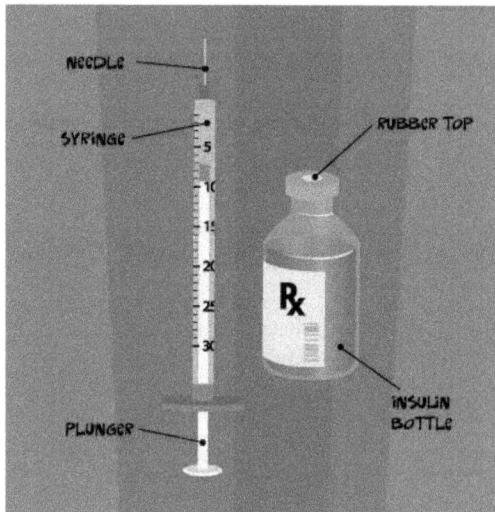

Insulin Injection Sites

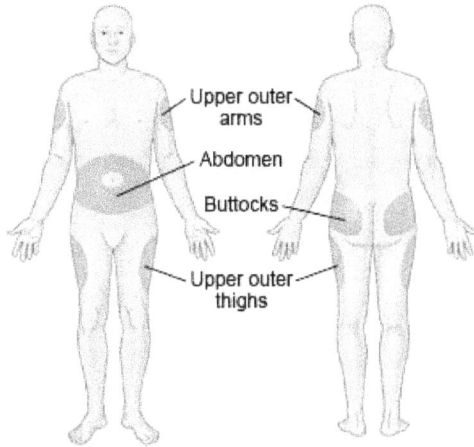

Insulin Injection

(3) Insulin Pumps:

An insulin siphon is a little gadget (somewhat bigger than a pack of cards) that conveys insulin into the layer of fat that sits just beneath the skin (subcutaneous tissue).

Since the insulin siphon remains associated with the body, it permits the wearer to alter the measure of insulin they take inside the press of a couple of catches whenever of the day or to program in a sequential pace of insulin conveyance to happen at a picked time, which can be when dozing.

An insulin siphon comprises of the principle siphon unit which holds an insulin supply that regularly holds somewhere in the range of 176 and 300 units of insulin. The store is connected to a long, slim bit of tubing with a needle or cannula toward one side. The tubing and the bit toward the end are known as the implantation set. Insulin siphon treatment is likewise alluded to as ceaseless subcutaneous insulin mixture treatment.

Around 1 out of 1,000 individuals with diabetes wear an insulin siphon.

Insulin siphons are electronic gadgets that are worn constantly and convey insulin into the fat layer underneath the skin by method for an adaptable plastic cylinder (like the "port" depicted previously). Insulin siphons are well known among the individuals who require various every day infusions of insulin. Sheltered and effective utilization of siphon requires extensive instruction and preparing, and their expense can be moderately high. Insulin siphons are not commonly utilized by the individuals who are new to insulin however can be a compelling alternative once you have more understanding.

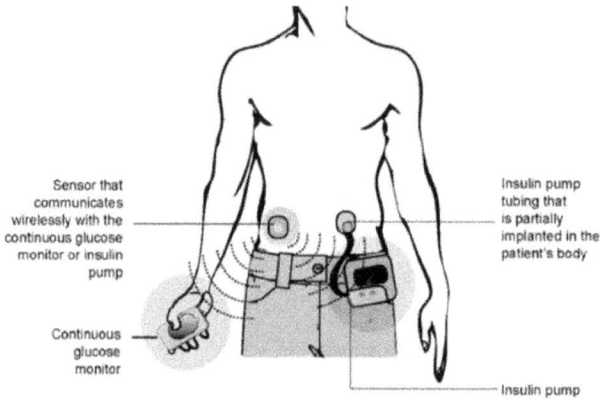

Picking an infusion gadget

The choice to utilize syringes or pens is an individual one. On the off chance that you have a chance to test both at your social insurance supplier's office, positively do as such. It is ideal to talk with your medicinal services supplier and check with your health care coverage to discover what is secured under

your arrangement. Most pens hold 300 units of insulin and permit conveyance of up to 60 to 80 units one after another. "Prefilled" expendable pens convey in single-unit increases. "Tough" pens use replaceable/insulin cartridges and may convey insulin in 1/2 unit increases. Pens can be utilized to convey an assortment of long-acting and quick acting insulin types, just as premixed insulin details. Dispensable syringes hold up to 100 units for each infusion. On the off chance that you choose to use syringes, select a sort that holds enough to cover your biggest portion with a little space to save. The markings on a syringe permit dosing in 2-unit, 1-unit, or 1/2-unit increases. When you have a size that addresses your issues, select a sort that permits you to portion as absolutely as could reasonably be expected.

The needles or syringes differ too. Syringe and pen needles as short as 4mm and as long as 12.7mm is accessible. Thickness is estimated in measure. The higher the check, the more slender the needle. Checks as high as 32 and as low as 28-measure can be acquired. When all is said in done, it is ideal to utilize the most limited, most slender (most elevated measure) needles accessible. Skin thickness doesn't fluctuate much from individual to individual. Regardless of whether you are overweight or fat, it is impossible that you will require a needle longer than 6mm. Needles that are too long may create difficult intramuscular infusions, with insulin engrossing quicker than it should.

Infusion Technique:

Strategy Is Everything When It Comes To Making Insulin Injections Easy.

To single Type of Insulin Into a Syringe:

Accumulate your insulin supplies:

Get your insulin vial and a new syringe. Check the insulin vial to ensure it is the correct sort of insulin and that there are no clusters or particles in it. Likewise, ensure the insulin isn't being utilized past its termination date.

Tenderly mix middle or premixed insulin:

Turn the container on its side and move it between the palms of your hands. Clear (quick acting, long-acting) insulin for the most part shouldn't be blended.

Set up the insulin bottle:

On the off chance that the insulin bottle is new, evacuate the top. It isn't important to wipe the highest point of the jug with liquor as long as it is spotless.

Maneuver air into the syringe:

Expel the top from the needle. Pull back the unclogger on the syringe to attract a measure of air that is equivalent to your insulin portion. The TIP of the dark unclogger ought to relate to the number on the syringe.

Infuse air into the vial:

Hold the syringe like a pencil and supplement the needle into the elastic plug on the highest point of the vial. Push the unclogger down until the entirety of the air is in the jug. This assists with keeping the perfect measure of weight in the contain and makes it simpler to draw the insulin.

Draw up the insulin into the syringe:

With the needle still in the vial, flip around the container and syringe (vial above syringe). Pull the unclogger to fill the syringe to the ideal sum.

Check the syringe for air bubbles:

In the event that you see any enormous air pockets, push the unclogger until the air is cleansed out of the syringe. Pull the unclogger withdraw to the ideal portion.

Expel the needle from the jug:

Be mindful so as to not let the needle contact anything until you are prepared to infuse it!

20.INFRARED LIGHT THERAPY FOR NEUROPATHY:

Diabetic Neuropathy

A few sorts of neuropathy (nerve harm) are brought about by diabetes. Find out about these diabetic neuropathies: fringe, autonomic, proximal, and central neuropathies. Clarifies what nerves are influenced in each kind of diabetic neuropathy.

Tolerant Guide to Treating High Cholesterol and Diabetes

Diabetic hyperlipidemia sounds somewhat scary, isn't that right? As we generally do here on EndocrineWeb, we're going to separate that idea for you, and that is the reason we've assembled this Patient Guide to Treating High Cholesterol and Diabetes.

Tolerant Guide to Insulin

The reason for the Patient Guide to Insulin is to teach patients, guardians, and parental figures about insulin treatment of diabetes. By investigating this data, you're making a significant move to find out about diabetes and how insulin controls the sickness to assist you with carrying on with a more advantageous life.

Tolerant Guide to Osteoporosis Prevention

In the event that you resemble numerous individuals, you may feel that osteoporosis—a condition set apart by low bone mineral thickness, which prompts brought down bone quality and an elevated danger of cracks—is something you won't need to stress over until some other time throughout everyday life.

Tolerant Guide to Easy Diabetic Recipes

Need some new thoughts for what to eat? We've assembled 5 tasty—and diabetes-accommodating—plans. Breakfast, lunch, supper—even an evening nibble and a yummy sweet. This current Patients' Guide will assist you with eating admirably throughout the day with our simple diabetic plans.

Thyroid Cancer Guide

A neck bump or knob is the most well-known side effect of thyroid malignancy. You may feel a protuberance, notice one side of your neck seems, by all accounts, to appear as something else, or your primary care physician may discover it during a normal assessment. On the off chance that the tumor is huge, it might cause neck or facial torment, brevity of breath, trouble gulping, hack irrelevant to a chilly, roughness or voice change.

Tolerant Guide to Managing Your Child's Type 1 Diabetes

This Patient Guide is structured particularly for guardians of kids with type 1 diabetes. Here, you'll find out about probably the most significant parts of dealing with your kid's condition.

✓ Treatment for neuropathy (Pain, consuming, pricking sensation in feet and legs).
✓ Infrared light builds the arrival of Nitric Oxide and results in positive bio cell reaction.
✓ Approved by USFDA (United States Food and Drug Administration) as the most recent treatment to expand the blood flow, diminish torment, muscle fit and solidness of legs.
✓ A positive outcome in 6 to 10 treatment sessions of 30 minutes span.
✓ It is a solitary, direct, non-obtrusive, effortless and viable approach to help with discomfort.

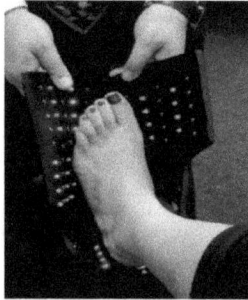

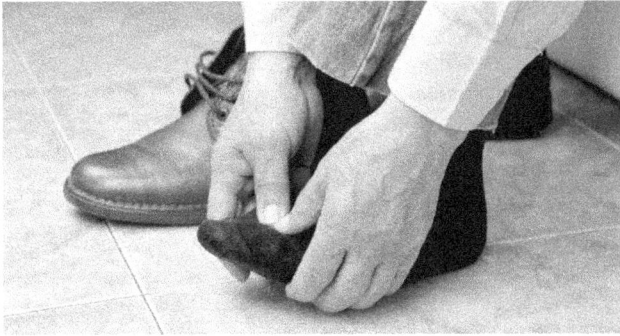

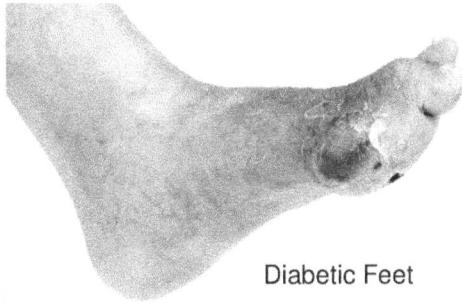

Diabetic Feet

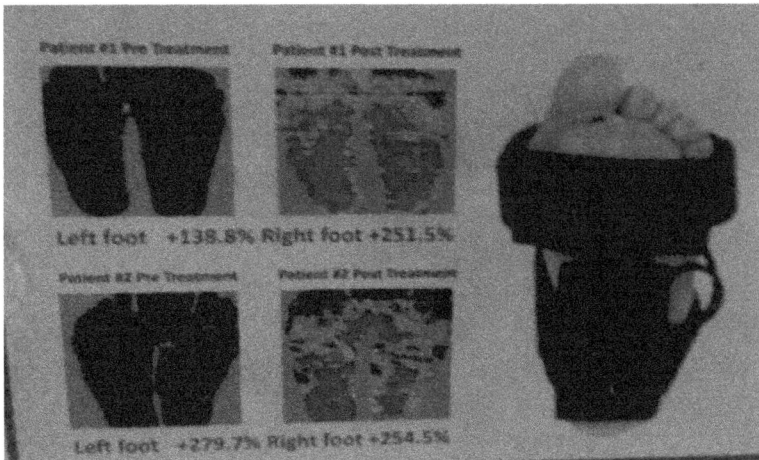

Patient #1 Pre Treatment   Patient #1 Post Treatment

Left foot   +138.8% Right foot +251.5%

Patient #2 Pre Treatment   Patient #2 Post Treatment

Left foot +279.7% Right foot +254.5%

Leg of the patient during pre treatment and post treatment

22. TREATMENT FOR CHRONIC HYPERGLYCEMIA ASSOCIATED INFECTIOUS DISEASES:

Patients with uncontrolled diabetes are viewed as immunosuppressed because of the negative impacts of raised blood sugars on the invulnerable framework. Hyperglycemia hinders by and large invulnerability through various systems. Interminable hyperglycemia in diabetes patients can prompt acidosis, which confines the movement of the invulnerable framework. The impacts of these progressions are endless supply of acidosis and hyperglycemia.

Ceaseless hyperglycemia eases back perfusion through veins, causing nerve harm as time advances. The skin, one of the key obstructions in natural insusceptibility, is never again skillful, yielding insurance against injury and aggravation. On account of weakened nerves in the skin, the host may not see injury to the skin until a contamination is available. Thus, skin and delicate tissue contaminations are conspicuous in diabetes patients with interminable hyperglycemia. Alongside poor administration of blood glucose, cellulitis and diabetic foot ulcers could recuperate more slow than wanted and progress to progressively serious conditions, for example, osteomyelitis. Such conditions must be dealt with quickly and effectively with antimicrobial treatment and other suitable enhancements of care (for example wound consideration and debridements). Harmed nerves are noted in the skin as well as in different regions of the body, for example, the urinary tract. With harm to the nerves in the urinary tract, pee maintenance will breed urinary tract contaminations.

In spite of the fact that the most well-known contaminations in diabetes patients include the skin and urinary tract, progressively serious diseases may emerge if blood sugars are not controlled. High glucose levels restrain and deregulate neutrophil combination, which is basic in the safe framework to assault a remote article. Cytosolic calcium in polymorphonuclear leukocytes (PMNs) augments inside seeing hyperglycemia and is alternately comparing to the occasion of phagocytosis in patients with type II diabetes. Significant levels of cytosolic calcium repress the blend of adenosine triphosphate (ATP), which is fundamental for phagocytosis. The capacity of PMN leukocytes to activate to the site of contamination and invigorate apoptosis is contrarily affected too.

On the off chance that the pathogen can attack the host without the help of the natural insusceptible framework, an expanded danger of contamination is normal. Hyperglycemia causes other bothersome changes in the capacity of the insusceptible framework, for example, diminished supplement reaction, leukocyte adherence and bactericidal movement.

Diseases:

Microorganisms' capacity to flourish within the sight of raised blood sugars initiates the insusceptible reaction to battle such contaminations. Also, a hyperglycemic state contrarily influences the body's capacity to react to antimicrobial treatment. Normal bacterial contaminations incorporate gram-negative life forms, for example, Pseudomonas aeruginosa, Klebsiella pneumonia, and E. coli. Gram-positive living beings, for example, Staphylococcus and Streptococcus are normal, too. Anaerobic creatures might be available also because of diminished blood and oxygen perfusion all through the veins for the combination of leukocytes. Different contaminations incorporate contagious diseases, for example, Candida and viral contaminations.

Head and Neck infections:

(1) Malignant Otitis Externa:

Etiology	Inflammation and damage at the base of the skull due to an untreated outer ear infection.
Source	*Pseudomonas aeruginosa* – most common organism.
Signs and Symptoms	Yellow-green drainage from the ear, odor, fever, deep inner ear pain.
Complications	Spread of infection throughout the body, Recurring infection, Brain and/or nerve damage, Osteomyelitis of temporal bone.
Antimicrobial Treatment	Cipro (Ciprofloxacin) 750 mg every 12 hours, oral route (or) 400 mg every 12 hours, intravenous route. Zosyn (Piperacillin/Tazobactam) 4g to 6 g

	each 4 to 6 hours, intravenous course. Timentin (Ticarcillin/Clavulanate Potassium) 3 g at regular intervals, intravenous course. Fortaz (Ceftazidime) 2 g at regular intervals, intravenous course. Maxime (Cefepime) 2 g every 12 hours, intravenous route.
Comments	In severe cases, Primaxin (Imipenem/cilastatin) may be used due to its pseudomonal coverage. Furthermore, aminoglycosides (for example gentamicin) in blend with antimicrobials with pseudomonal inclusion might be utilized. Ciprofloxacin resistant strands of *Pseudomonas* do not increase morbidity or mortality.

(2) Rhinocerebral Mucormycosis:

Etiology	Initially presents itself as an acute sinus infection. Caused by the inhalation of fungal spores which can move quickly to the brain if not treated promptly.
Source	Saprophytic aerobic fungi found in soil and bread mold.
Signs and Symptoms	Headache, Nausea, vomiting, fever and lethargy. Inflammation. Facial: Weakness, numbness & pain.

	Nasal: Pale or gray Necrotizing (black) areas in the face, pus drainage.
	Ocular: Fixed pupil, Nystagmus, Blindness.
	Nerves: Altered mental status, Dizziness & unsteady gait.
	Negative effects of the following cranial nerves: II, III, IV, V, VI, & VII Cerebral edema.
Complications	Failure of prompt treatment may progress the condition to a coma or stroke.
Antimicrobial Treatment	First-line therapy: Debridement Amphotericin B (weight-based dose). Elective treatment: Noxafil (Posaconazole) 400 mg twice day by day, oral course (suspension).
Comments	Nephrotoxicity (associated with Amphotericin B; consider lipid-based formulation). Achievement of steady-state with posaconazole occurs in 1 week; it should not be considered as initial therapy. While providing antifungal treatment, the underlying cause of the compromised immune system must be addressed (i.e. hyperglycemia). The duration of treatment is dependent on the patient's response to therapy.

Gastrointestinal and Liver infections:

(1) Emphysematous Cholecystitis:

Etiology	Discovery of gas in gallbladder lumen, wall or surrounding tissues. Gallstones = ~50% of all cases
Source	Polymicrobial infection: gram-positive, gram-negative and anaerobes.
Signs and Symptoms	Right upper quadrant pain not related to physical activity; may radiate. Fever, Absent bowel sounds.
Complications	Perforated gallbladder, Septic shock.
Antimicrobial Treatment	Broad-spectrum antibiotics: Example(s): Zosyn, Unasyn, Primaxin.
Comments	Antimicrobial combinations may be used and should possess gram-positive, pseudomonal, and anaerobic coverage.

Skin and Soft tissues infections:

(1) SSTI (Skin and Soft Tissue Infections):

Etiology	Inflammation or wounds.
Source	Gram-positive MRSA (Methicillin-Resistant Staphylococcus aureus), Polymicrobial contamination.
Signs and Symptoms	Inflammation or wounds that neglect to recuperate appropriately.
Complications	Development into increasingly extreme conditions, for example, osteomyelitis or necrotizing fasciitis.
Antimicrobial Treatment	MSSA (Methicillin Sensitive Staphylococcus aureus) SSTIs: Nafcillin, Oxacillin, Dicloxacillin, Cefazolin.

	CA-MRSA(Community Associated MRSA) SSTIs: Vancomycin.
	Zyvox (Linezolid) 600 mg like clockwork, intravenous or oral course.
	Cleocin (Clindamycin) 600 mg/kg like clockwork, intravenous course (or) 300-450 mg multiple times every day, oral course.
	Cubicin (Daptomycin) 4 mg/kg consistently, intravenous course.
	Doxycycline 100 mg twice day by day, oral course.
	Bactrim (TMP-SMZ) 1-2 twofold quality tablets twice day by day, oral course.
Comments	De-heighten antimicrobial when suitable. Vancomycin trough ranges: 10-15 mg/L for minor diseases, 15-20 mg/L for extreme contaminations.

(2) Diabetic Foot Infections:

Etiology	Lack of blood flow due to chronic hyperglycemia, peripheral vascular disease, and neuropathy. Polymicrobial infection.
Source	Polymicrobial infection including *S. aureus*, *Streptococcus* & *P. aeruginosa*
Signs and Symptoms	Tachycardia, Hypotension, Pain, Fever, Chills, Purulent discharge, Erythema.
Complications	Osteomyelitis, Necrotizing fasciitis, Amputation.

Antimicrobial Treatment	Mild treatment - Dicloxacillin, Keflex (Cephalexin), Levaquin (Levofloxacin), Augmentin (Amoxicillin/ clavulanate), Doxycycline, Bactrim DS (TMP-SMZ). Moderate- Severe: Levaquin (Levofloxacin), Rocephin (Ceftriaxone), Unasyn (Ampicillin-Sulbactam), Avelox (Moxifloxacin), Invanz (Ertapenem), Tygacil (Tygecycline), Levaquin or Cipro + Clindamycin, Vancomycin, Zosyn (Piperacillintazobactam), Cubicin (Daptomycin), Fortaz (Ceftazidime), Maxipime (Cefepime).
Comments	Wound care & debridement play a major role in the healing process of these infections. De-escalate antimicrobial therapy when appropriate. Vancomycin trough range: 15-20 mg/L.

(3) Necrotizing Fasciitis:

Etiology	Lethal infection due to untreated wounds.
Source	Polymicrobial infection including anaerobes.
Signs and Symptoms	Skin necrosis, Blisters, Gas in soft tissue, Spread of necrotic tissue in spite of antibiotics.
Complications	Amputation, Sepsis.
Antimicrobial Treatment	Anti-pseudomonal fluoroquinolone i.e. Cipro Zosyn 4.5 grams every 6 hours, intravenous route. Clindamycin 600-600 mg every 8 hours,

	intravenous route.
	Vancomycin 15-20 mg/kg every 12 hours, intravenous route.
	Primaxin 1 g every 6-8 hours, intravenous route.
	Merrem (Meropenem) 1g every 8 hours, intravenous route.
	Fortaz 2 g at regular intervals, intravenous course + Flagyl 500 mg like clockwork, intravenous course (or) Clindamycin (see portion above).
	Aminoglycosides.
Comments	Wound care & debridement play a major role in the healing process of these infections. Combination therapy may be used to effectively treat an infection. Vancomycin trough range: 15-20 mg/L.

(4) Bullous diabeticorum:

Etiology	Unknown
Source	Not Applicable
Signs and Symptoms	Blisters
Complications	Development of osteomyelitis, Amputation.
Antimicrobial Treatment	Not Applicable
Comments	Spontaneous healing in 2- 6 weeks.

Bone infections:

(1) Osteomyelitis:

Etiology	Untreated infection that has spread to the bone.
Source	*S. aureus*, Gram-negative bacilli, Polymicrobial infection.
Signs and Symptoms	Localized pain, Tenderness in the infected area, Swelling, fever, Erythema.
Complications	Amputation, Sepsis.
Antimicrobial Treatment	Augmentin 875 mg twice daily, oral route. Zosyn 3.375 g every 6 hours, intravenous route. Unasyn 3 g every 6 hours, intravenous route. Timentin 3.1 g every 6 hours, intravenous route. Clindamycin 600 mg like clockwork, intravenous course or oral course + Cipro 750 mg oral course (or) 400 mg at regular intervals, intravenous course (or) Levaquin750 mg day by day, oral course + Vancomycin 15mg/kg like clockwork, intravenous course if MRSA is suspected or affirmed.
Comments	Wound care & debridement play a major role in the healing process of these infections. Treatment should be a minimum of 6 weeks. Vancomycin trough range: 15-20 mg/L.

Urinary Tract infections:

(1) Pyelonephritis:

Etiology	Bacteria in the urinary tract/Upper urinary tract disease influencing the kidneys.
Source	Gram-negative living beings E. Coli, P. mirabilis, P. aeruginosa, and so forth and Yeast. At times, polymicrobial disease is available.
Signs and Symptoms	Dysuria, Flank torment and Abdominal uneasiness.
Complications	Toxic fever, Chills, Dry mucous layers, Tachycardia.
Antimicrobial Treatment	Fluoroquinolones. Cipro (Ciprofloxacin) 500 mg twice every day, oral course. Levaquin (Levofloxacin) 750 mg every day, oral course. In the event that oral course is heinous, think about the accompanying choices of treatment: Cipro or Levaquin IV Zosyn (Piperacillin – tazobactam) 3.375 mg at regular intervals, intravenous course. Primaxin (Imipenem-Cilastatin) 500 mg at regular intervals, intravenous course. Merrem (Meropenem) 1 g at regular intervals, intravenous course. Ampicillin 1-2 g at regular intervals + Gentamicin 2mg/kg/portion like clockwork, intravenous course.

Comments	Longer span of treatment (7-14 days).
	Levaquin = 5 days of treatment.
	Second-line treatment: Fortaz (Ceftazidime) 500 mg each 8-12 hours, intravenous course for 10 days.
	Maxime (Cefepime) 2 g at regular intervals, intravenous course for 10 days.
	Bactrim DS/Septra DS might be considered.

23.-MYTHS AND FACTS

Diabetes is an annoyance yet not genuine

Diabetes causes a greater number of passings in a year than bosom malignant growth and AIDS joined. Having diabetes about copies your opportunity of having a cardiovascular failure. 66% of diabetes patients bite the dust rashly from stroke or coronary illness. The future of an individual with diabetes is from five to ten years shorter than other people's. Fortunately great diabetes control can lessen your dangers for diabetes inconveniences.

Eating an excess of sugar causes diabetes

Type 1 diabetes is brought about by hereditary qualities and obscure elements that trigger the beginning of the illness and type 2 diabetes is brought about by hereditary qualities and way of life factors.

An individual with type 1 diabetes built up the infection on the grounds that their insusceptible framework wrecked the insulin-creating beta cells. Type 2 diabetes is created if there is a background marked by diabetes in the family.

Overweight/Obese expands the danger of creating type 2 diabetes and an eating routine high in calories from any source adds to weight gain. Research has demonstrated that drinking sugary beverages is connected to type 2 diabetes.

The American Diabetes Association suggests that individuals ought to keep away from the admission of sugar-improved refreshments to help forestall diabetes. Sugar-improved refreshments incorporate refreshments like normal pop, fruit juice and beverages, caffeinated drinks, sports drinks, improved tea and other sugary beverages. These beverages will raise blood glucose and can give a few hundred calories in only one serving.

Note: Just one 12-ounce container of normal soft drink has around 150 calories and 40 grams of starch. This is a similar measure of starch in 10 teaspoons of sugar.

One cup of fruit juice and other sugary natural product drinks have around 100 calories (or more) and 30 grams of starch.

Children can exceed diabetes

About all kids with diabetes have type 1 and insulin-creating beta cells in the pancreas have been pulverized. These never returned. Kids with type 1 diabetes should take insulin for the remainder of their lives except if a fix is discovered one day.

Fat individuals consistently create type 2 diabetes

Being overweight or hefty raises the danger of getting diabetic, they are hazard factors yet don't imply that a corpulent individual will get diabetic. Numerous individuals with type 2 diabetes were rarely overweight. Most of overweight individuals don't create type 2 diabetes.

Diabetic individuals ought not work out

Exercise is significant for diabetic individuals, all things considered for every other person. Exercise assists with overseeing body weight, improves cardiovascular wellbeing, improves state of mind, assists blood with sugaring control and eases pressure. Patients ought to counsel and talk about the activity with their primary care physician first.

Diabetic individuals know when their glucose levels are high or low

High or low glucose levels may cause a few side effects, for example, shortcoming, weakness and extraordinary thirst. Glucose levels can vacillate and a great deal of side effects can be felt. The best way to make certain about your glucose levels is to test them routinely. Scientists from the University of Copenhagen, Denmark indicated that even slight ascents in blood-glucose levels altogether raise the danger of ischemic coronary illness.

People with diabetes ought to eat extraordinary diabetic nourishments

A sound supper plan for individuals with diabetes is commonly equivalent to a solid eating routine for anybody. Suppers ought to contain a lot of vegetables, organic product, entire grains and they ought to be low in salt and sugar and immersed or trans fat. Diabetic and "dietetic" nourishments by and large offer no unique advantage. The vast majority of them despite everything raise blood glucose levels, are generally increasingly costly and can likewise have a diuretic impact on the off chance that they contain sugar liquor.

Diabetics can't eat bread, potatoes or pasta

Individuals with diabetes can eat dull nourishments. Boring nourishments can be a piece of a solid supper plan, yet to watch out for the size of the parts. Entire grain bread, oats, pasta, rice and dull vegetables like potatoes, yams, peas and corn can be remembered for your dinners and tidbits. Notwithstanding these dull nourishments, organic products, beans, milk, yogurt, and desserts are likewise wellsprings of sugars that you have to include in your feast plan. Be that as it may, you may require more or less starches at suppers relying upon how you deal with your diabetes.

Diabetic individuals can't eat desserts or chocolates

Whenever eaten as a major aspect of a sound feast plan or joined with exercise, desserts and pastries can be eaten by diabetic individuals. They can be taken in a little segment yet the principle spotlight ought to be on your supper with restorative nourishments.

The organic product is sound nourishment. Along these lines, it is alright to take more

The organic product is sound nourishment. It contains more fiber and loads of nutrients and minerals. Since natural products contain sugars and they must be remembered for your supper plan. Counsel your dietitian about the sum, recurrence and kinds of organic products that ought to be taken.

Diabetes can be transmitted

No. Diabetes can't be transmitted starting with one individual then onto the next individual. It isn't irresistible or infectious. A parent may pass on, through their qualities to their posterity, higher vulnerability to building up the infection.

Only more seasoned individuals create type 2 diabetes

Things are evolving. A developing number of youngsters and adolescents are creating type 2 diabetes. Specialists state this is connected to the blast in youth weight rates, terrible eating routine, and physical latency.

✓ Diabetic individuals need to go on insulin-this signifies "their diabetes is extreme"

Individuals take insulin when diet alone or diet with oral or non-insulin injectable diabetes drugs don't give adequate diabetes control, that's it in a nutshell. Insulin helps in diabetes control. It doesn't normally have anything to do with the seriousness of the malady.

✓ Diabetic individuals are bound to get colds and different ailments

A diabetic individual with great diabetes control is not any more liable to turn out to be sick with a cold or something different than others. Be that as it may, when a diabetic comes down with a bug, their diabetes gets more earnestly to control, so they have a higher danger of inconveniences.

24. QUICK FACTS ON DIABETES

➤ Diabetes is a long haul condition that causes high glucose levels.

➤ In 2012, an expected 1.5 million passings were legitimately brought about by diabetes.

➤ In 2013 it was assessed that more than 382 million individuals all through the world had diabetes (William's reading material of endocrinology).

➤ In 2014 the worldwide predominance of diabetes was assessed to be 9% among grown-ups matured 18+ years.

➤ More than 80% of diabetes passings happen in low-and center salary nations.

➤ Type 1 Diabetes - the body doesn't create insulin. Around 10% of each and every one diabetes cases are type 1.

➤ Type 2 Diabetes - the body doesn't create enough insulin for legitimate capacity. Roughly 90% of all instances of diabetes overall are of this sort.

- Gestational Diabetes - This sort influences females during pregnancy.
- The most normal diabetes manifestations incorporate continuous pee, extraordinary thirst and yearning, weight increase, bizarre weight reduction, exhaustion, cuts and wounds that don't mend, male sexual brokenness, deadness and shivering in hands and feet.
- If you have Type 1 and follow a good dieting arrangement, do satisfactory exercise and take insulin, you can have an ordinary existence.
- Type 2 patients need to eat soundly, be genuinely dynamic and test their blood glucose. They may likewise need to take oral medicine, and additionally insulin to control blood glucose levels.
- As the danger of cardiovascular illness is a lot higher for a diabetic, it is urgent that circulatory strain and cholesterol levels are checked consistently.
- As smoking may seriously affect cardiovascular wellbeing, diabetics should quit smoking.
- Hypoglycemia - Low blood glucose - can badly affect the patient. Hyperglycemia - when blood glucose is excessively high - it can likewise badly affect the patient.
- Insulin-delivering cells offer trust in individuals with type 1 diabetes.
- Prolonged sitting connected to expanded danger of non-alcoholic greasy liver malady.
- Long daytime sluggishness could build the danger of diabetes.
- Sugary drinks raise the danger of coronary episode and coronary illness more than by a third.
- Blood pressure drug before bed could bring down the danger of diabetes.
- Childhood stress may raise the danger of diabetes and coronary illness in adulthood.
- Smoking and detached smoking connected to a more serious danger of type 2 diabetes.
- A sound eating routine, standard physical movement, keeping up typical body weight and maintaining a strategic distance from tobacco use can forestall or defer the beginning of type 2 diabetes.
- WHO ventures that diabetes will be the seventh driving reason for death in 2030.

25. GLOSSARY

A sleeping disorder - It is a rest issue. Individuals have the failure to rest.

Acidosis – Excessive corrosiveness in the blood and other body tissues. It is caused either by an excess of corrosive in the blood/loss of bicarbonate from the blood called metabolic acidosis or via carbon dioxide development in the blood that outcomes from poor lung work/moderate breathing called respiratory acidosis.

Adulthood - It is where individual or other living being has arrived at sexual development. i.e., the presence of optional sex attributes, for example, discharge in men, feminine cycle in ladies and pubic hair in both genders.

Ailing health - It is a condition that outcomes from eating an eating routine where supplements are either insufficient or are an excessive amount of with the end goal that the eating regimen messes wellbeing up. It might include calories, protein, starches, nutrients or minerals. Insufficient supplements are called undernutrition while a lot of is called overnutrition.

Alzheimer's malady – (The name, Alzheimer's, originates from the German specialist, Alois Alzheimer, who previously noticed the illness). Alzheimer's is a type of dementia that has been seen as firmly connected with type 2 diabetes and contemplated 1 of every 15 individuals beyond 65 years old. Alzheimer's is portrayed by perplexity and loss of memory. This is commonly analyzed further down the road. The malady is expedited by harm to nerves and cells in the mind, with the early indications of conspicuous by disarray, discourse challenges and carelessness.

Autoantibodies - A neutralizer that is a sort of protein created by the safe framework that is coordinated against at least one of the person's own proteins. Numerous immune system maladies are brought about by such autoantibodies. Model: Graves' infection - Thyroid autoantibodies (TSHR-Ab) that initiate the TSH-receptor (TSHR).

Autoimmunity - Arrangement of resistant reactions of a living being against its own cell and tissues. Any illness that outcomes from such an irregular insusceptible reaction is known as an immune system malady. Model: Diabetes Mellitus Type 1.

Beta cells (β cells) - These are a kind of cells found in the pancreatic islets. They compose up 65-80% of the cells inside islets. The essential capacity of these cells is to store and discharge insulin.

Cancer prevention agent - It is a particle that represses the oxidation of different atoms. Oxidation is a compound reaction that can make free radicals, provoking chain reactions that may hurt cells.

Cardiomyopathy - It is a heart muscle ailment. The heart muscle gets expanded, thick or unbending. In unusual cases, the muscle tissue within the heart is supplanted with scar tissue. The debilitating of the heart prompts cardiovascular breakdown or unpredictable pulses called arrhythmias.

Cardiovascular ailment – Heart infection is an inconvenience that may influence individuals with diabetes if their condition isn't overseen well for a drawn out timeframe. Coronary illness is perceived to be the reason for death for 80% of individuals with diabetes, in any case, respiratory failures are to a great extent preventable. Both sort 1 and type 2 diabetics are at more serious danger of creating coronary illness. The regular side effects of coronary illness are torment in the chest, shy of breath, unpredictable heartbeat and growing of lower legs.

Cerebrum mist - Feelings of mental perplexity or absence of mental lucidity.

Clogging - A condition where there is trouble in discharging the insides, ordinarily connected with solidified defecation. It is a typical reason for agonizing crap.

Coenzyme Q10 - Coenzyme Q10 (CoQ10) is a characteristic cell reinforcement incorporated by the body, found in numerous nourishments and accessible as an enhancement. It comes in two structures: ubiquinol, the dynamic cell reinforcement structure and ubiquinone, the oxidized structure, which the body incompletely changes over to ubiquinol. It is said to help cardiovascular breakdown just as malignant growth, solid dystrophy and periodontal ailment.

Consideration Deficit-Hyperactivity Disorder (ADHD) - National Institute of Mental Health (NIMH) characterizes ADHD as a cerebrum issue set apart by a continuous example of obliviousness as well as hyperactivity, impulsivity that meddles with working or advancement. It is more typical in guys than in females. The hazard components may incorporate qualities; cigarette smoking, liquor drinking and introduction to ecological poisons during pregnancy, and so forth.

Constant weakness disorder (CFS) - It is a genuine ailment that can cause long haul ailment and incapacity, yet numerous individuals, especially youngsters and youngsters - improve after some time. It causes tireless weariness (fatigue) that influences regular day to day existence and doesn't leave with rest or rest. It is otherwise called ME (myalgic encephalomyelitis).

Coronary episode - A cardiovascular failure happens when the progression of oxygen-rich blood to an area of heart muscle unexpectedly gets blocked and the heart can't get oxygen. On the off chance that blood stream isn't reestablished rapidly, the area of the heart muscle starts to kick the bucket. Respiratory failures regularly happen because of coronary illness (CHD), likewise called coronary conduit malady. CHD is a condition where a waxy substance called plaque develops inside the coronary supply routes. These veins supply oxygen-rich blood to the heart.

Cortisol - It is a steroid hormone created in people by the zona fasciculate of the adrenal cortex inside the adrenal organ. It capacities to expand glucose through gluconeogenesis, to smother the resistant framework and to help in the digestion of fat, protein and sugars.

Craving – It is the longing to eat nourishment, in some cases because of yearning. It exists in all higher living things. To keep up the metabolic needs of the body, it serves to direct more vitality consumption.

Cytomegalovirus (CMV) - It is gotten from the Greek word, 'cyto' signifies "cell" and 'megalo' signifies "huge". It is a class of infections that has a place with the family Herpesviridae. The species that contaminates people is ordinarily known as human CMV (HCMV) or human herpesvirus-5 (HHV-5). Illnesses related with HHV-5 incorporate mononucleosis and pneumonia.

Deadness - It is lost sensation or feeling in a piece of the human body. It is an irregular sensation regularly felt in fingers, hands, feet, arms or legs. Deadness can happen along a solitary nerve, on one side of the body, or it might happen evenly, on the two sides of the body. There are numerous causes remembering sitting or representing a similar situation for quite a while, harming a nerve, absence of Vitamin B12, radiation treatment, creature nibbles, utilization of specific prescriptions, diabetes, headaches, stroke, seizures, an underactive thyroid, and so on.,

Deferasirox – Oral iron chelator. Its principle use is to diminish ceaseless iron over-burden in patients who are getting long haul blood transfusions for conditions, for example, beta-thalassemia and other constant anemias. It is the primary oral medicine endorsed in the USA for this reason.

Dermatitis - It is the irritation of the skin. Side effects incorporate bothersome, red and dry skin. It is most usually found in youngsters, despite the fact that grown-ups can get it. It is additionally called atopic dermatitis and is treated with oral meds, steroid creams and light treatment.

Development Onset Diabetes of the Young (MODY) - Rare type of diabetes which is not quite the same as both sort 1 and type 2 diabetes. It is brought about by a transformation (or change) in a solitary quality. On the off chance that a parent has this quality transformation, any youngster they have has a half possibility of acquiring it from them.

Diet - In sustenance, diet is the total of nourishment devoured by an individual. It frequently suggests the utilization of explicit admission of nourishment for wellbeing or weight-the board reasons. Singular dietary decisions might be pretty much sound.

Disorder X - It is a typical term utilized for a newfound gathering of manifestations. It might allude to heart disorder X (chest torment with signs related with diminished blood stream to heart tissue however with ordinary coronary veins), metabolic disorder (related with the danger of creating cardiovascular sickness and diabetes), Turner disorder (individual has a solitary X chromosome) and intense radiation disorder (assortment of wellbeing impacts that are available inside 24 hours of introduction to high measures of ionizing radiation).

Diverticulosis - It is the state of having diverticula (outpouching of an empty or a liquid filled structure in the body) in the colon, which are out stashing of the colonic mucosa and submucosa through shortcomings of muscle layers in the colon divider. Diverticular illness happens when diverticula become excited or drain.

Endometrial malignant growth – It is an Uterine disease. (The endometrium is the piece of the uterus - the empty strong organ which holds and secures a developing child during pregnancy). It is a typical type of malignancy in ladies which influences the female conceptive framework. It is increasingly regular in more established ladies beyond 50 years old, and like different types of disease, can be a confusion of long haul diabetes.

Epilepsy - It is a gathering of neurological illnesses portrayed by epileptic seizures. These seizures may introduce in a few different ways relying upon the piece of the cerebrum in question and the individual's age.

Epileptic seizures - It is a concise scene of signs or side effects because of unusual exorbitant or cadenced or redundant neural action in the focal sensory system (cerebrum and spinal string).

Erectile brokenness (Impotence) – It is sexual brokenness depicted by the inability to make or keep up an erection of the penis during sexual development in individuals.Causes are typically medicinal yet can likewise be mental. One of the elements prompting erectile brokenness are diabetes mellitus (causing neuropathy). Average first-line treatment of erectile brokenness includes the utilization of meds called PDE-5 inhibitors (phosphodiesterase type 5 inhibitor) including the notable medication sildenafil (Viagra).

Extremely Low-Calorie Diet (VLCD) - It is characterized as an eating regimen of 800 kcal (3300 kJ) every day or less.

Fart – It is gotten from the Latin word "flatus" which signifies "a blowing, a flatulating". It is the amassing of gas in the nutritious trench. The logical investigation of this territory of medication is named flatology.

Fat - It is one of the three fundamental macronutrients. It is otherwise called triglycerides, are esters of three unsaturated fat chains and liquor glycerol. They are commonly hydrophobic and are dissolvable in natural solvents and insoluble in water.

Feed fever (unfavorably susceptible rhinitis) - It creates when the body's invulnerable framework gets sharpened and blows up to something in the condition that commonly causes no issue in the vast majority. A couple of indications are runny nose; bothersome eyes, mouth or skin; sniffling and weariness.

Fiber/Fiber - It is from the Latin word "fibra". It is a characteristic or manufactured substance that is fundamentally longer than it is wide. Fiber is a significant piece of a sound adjusted eating regimen. It can help forestall coronary illness, diabetes, weight addition and a few tumors and can likewise improve stomach related wellbeing. Fiber is just found in nourishments that originate from plants. Nourishments, for example, meat, fish and dairy items don't contain any fiber.

Fibrosis - The advancement of sinewy connective tissue as a reparative reaction to damage or harm. It might allude to the connective tissue affidavit that happens as a component of ordinary recuperating or to the overabundance tissue testimony that happens as a neurotic procedure. At the point when fibrosis happens because of damage, the expression "scarring" is utilized. Model: Pulmonary fibrosis, Liver cirrhosis, Cardiac fibrosis.

FPG - It is a Fasting Plasma Glucose Test. It is a blood test that decides the measure of glucose (sugar) in the blood after a medium-term quick (not eating for in any event 8 hours). A fasting blood glucose level somewhere in the range of 100 and 125 mg/dl implies an individual has pre-diabetes. A fasting blood glucose level of 126 mg/dl or higher methods an individual has diabetes.

Fundamental Sclerosis - It is an immune system malady of the connective tissue. It is portrayed by changes in the surface and presence of the skin. This is because of expanded collagen (part of connective tissue) generation. It can influence veins, muscles, heart, lungs, kidneys and stomach related framework. It is otherwise called Systemic Scleroderma.

Gangrene – It is a non-transferable infection. It is a limited passing and deterioration of body tissues, coming about because of impeded dissemination or bacterial disease. Diabetes and long haul smoking increment the danger of experiencing gangrene.

Gastrin - It is a direct peptide hormone created by G cells of the duodenum and in the pyloric antrum of the stomach. It is discharged into the circulation system. It invigorates the emission of gastric corrosive (HCl) by the parietal cells of the stomach and helps in gastric motility.

Gastroparesis – It is gotten from the Greek word, 'gastro' signifies "stomach" and 'paresis' signifies "halfway loss of motion". It is otherwise called postponed gastric exhausting. It is a confusion that eases back or prevents the development of nourishment from the stomach to the small digestive tract. It can happen when the vagus nerve (controls the stomach muscles) is harmed by disease or damage and the stomach muscles quit working regularly.

Glaucoma – It is a condition that makes harm the eye's optic nerve and deteriorates after some time. Glaucoma is connected with higher-than-conventional load inside the eye, a condition called visual hypertension. In case untreated or uncontrolled, glaucoma first causes periphery vision mishap and at last can provoke visual impedance.

Glucose - Glucose is the most generally utilized aldohexose in living beings. Glucose is a universal fuel in science. It is utilized as a vitality source in many creatures, from microbes to people, through either high-impact breath, anaerobic breath or maturation.

Glyc(a)emic Index - A number that speaks to the overall capacity of a starch nourishment to build the degree of glucose in the blood.

Glyc(a)emic Load - A number that assessments how much the nourishment will raise a person's blood glucose level in the wake of eating eat. GL = GI * Carbohydrate/100.

Gout - It is a sort of joint inflammation. It can cause an assault of abrupt consuming agony, firmness, and growing in a joint, typically a major toe. These assaults can occur again and again except if gout is dealt with. After some time, they can hurt joints, ligaments, and different tissues. It is generally basic in men. It is brought about by an excessive amount of uric corrosive in the blood. At the point when uric corrosive levels in the blood are excessively high, the uric corrosive may shape hard gems in joints.

Harm - It is gotten from the Latin word, 'male' signifying "seriously" and 'gnus' signifying "conceived". It is the propensity of an ailment to turn out to be dynamically more terrible.

Hemochromatosis – It is an iron issue wherein the body basically stacks an excessive amount of iron. This activity is hereditary and the overabundance iron, whenever left untreated, can harm joints, organs, and in the long run be deadly. Undiscovered and untreated hemochromatosis expands the hazard for maladies and conditions, for example, diabetes mellitus, coronary failure, joint pain, liver cirrhosis, weakness, fruitlessness, hypothyroidism, and soon.,

Hemorrhoids - They are developed and swollen veins situated in the lower some portion of the rectum and the butt. The veins become swollen because of expanded weight inside them. They are normally brought about by expanded weight inside the lower guts. The different sorts are Internal hemorrhoids, External hemorrhoids and thrombosed outside hemorrhoids.

Hepatic cirrhosis - Cirrhosis is the extreme scarring of the liver and poor liver capacity seen at the terminal phases of ceaseless liver infection. The scarring is frequently brought about by long haul introduction to poisons, for example, liquor or viral diseases. As per the National Institutes of Health, cirrhosis is the twelfth driving reason for death by ailment.

HHNS - It is Hyperosmolar Hyperglycemic Nonketotic Syndrome. It is a genuine condition most as often as possible seen in more seasoned people. HHNS can happen to individuals with either type 1 or type 2 diabetes that isn't being controlled appropriately, however it happens all the more regularly in individuals with type 2.

Hypertension (HTN or HT) – It is a long haul ailment where the pulse in the corridors is tirelessly raised. It is otherwise called hypertension (HBP) higher than 140 more than 90 mmHg (millimeters of mercury). It is a significant hazard factor of coronary conduit ailment, stroke, cardiovascular breakdown, vision misfortune and ceaseless kidney malady.

IDDM - It is Insulin - Dependent Diabetes Mellitus, otherwise called Diabetes mellitus type 1. It is an immune system malady bringing about the decimation of insulin-creating beta cells in the pancreas. The consequent absence of insulin prompts expanded glucose in blood and pee. Side effects are visit pee, expanded thirst, expanded craving and weight reduction.

Idiopathic - It is gotten from the Greek word, 'idios' signifies "one's own", 'tenderness' signifies "languishing". Idiopathy implies roughly "an infection of its own sort". For instance, intense idiopathic polyneuritis, idiopathic scoliosis, diffuse idiopathic skeletal hyperostosis.

IGT - It is Impaired Glucose Tolerance, A pre-diabetic condition of hyperglycemia that is related with insulin obstruction and an expanded danger of cardiovascular pathology. It might go before type 2 diabetes mellitus for a long time. It is additionally a hazard factor for mortality.

Injury - It is physical damage or harm to a natural life form from an outer source. Insulin - It is gotten from Latin, 'insula' signifies "island". It is a peptide hormone made by the pancreas that permits the body to utilize sugar (glucose) from starches in the nourishment that we eat for vitality or to store glucose for sometime later. Insulin assists keeps with blooding sugar level from getting excessively high (hyperglycemia) or excessively low (hypoglycemia).

Insulin obstruction - When insulin levels are adequately high over a drawn out timeframe making the body's own affectability the hormone to be decreased. Side effects are dormancy, hunger, hypertension and cerebrum mist (sentiments of mental perplexity).

Ischaemic (Ischemic) heart illnesses (IHD) – It is otherwise called Coronary course infection (CAD). Ischemia implies a "decreased blood supply". It is a malady described by the diminished blood supply to the heart. The main sign is once in a while a coronary episode. Different entanglements incorporate cardiovascular breakdown or a sporadic heartbeat.

Ketoacidosis – It is a metabolic state related with high centralizations of ketone bodies, shaped by the breakdown of unsaturated fats and the deamination of amino acids. In ketoacidosis, the body neglects to sufficiently control ketone generation causing such an extreme gathering of keto acids that the pH of the blood is generously diminished. In extraordinary cases, ketoacidosis can be lethal.

Ketogenic Diet - The eating regimen depends on the standards of low sugar, high protein and high fat.

Ketosis – Ketosis is an ordinary metabolic procedure, something your body does to continue working. At the point when it needs more sugars from nourishment for your cells to consume for vitality, it consumes fat. As a feature of this procedure, it makes ketones. Ketosis can become risky when ketones develop. Significant levels lead to drying out and change the synthetic parity of the blood.

LCHF- Abstains from food (Low Carbohydrate High Fat weight control plans) - The eating routine which proposes eating high fat and low sugar nourishments.

Leptin - In Greek 'leptos' signifies "meager". It is the "starvation hormone". It is a hormone made by fat cells that assists with controlling vitality balance by restraining hunger. Leptin is contradicted by the activities of the hormone ghrelin, the "hunger hormone".

Liver - It is an enormous, substantial organ that sits on the correct side of the paunch. Weighing around 3 pounds, the liver is rosy darker in shading and feels rubbery to the touch. Regularly we can't feel the liver, since it's secured by the rib confine. It has two enormous areas, the privilege and the left projections. Its principle work is to channel the blood originating from the stomach related tract, before passing it to the remainder of the body.

Looseness of the bowels - passing free, watery stools multiple times each day. It is ordinarily experienced because of gastroenteritis however may likewise be brought about by explicit drug including statins and metformin. The normal causes are nourishment bigotries, (for example, lactose or gluten prejudice), entrail contamination and drinking a lot of espresso or liquor. On the off chance that looseness of the bowels perseveres longer, it is joined by different side effects, for example, fever, blood in your stools, heaving and unexplained weight reduction.

Low Carbohydrate eats less - The American Academy of Family Physicians characterizes low sugar slims down as diets that confine admission of starch to 20 to 60 grams for every day, normally under 20% of caloric admission.

Low-Calorie consumes less calories - It gives an objective admission of calories every day. It gives a relentless method to accomplish weight reduction.

Low-Fat eating regimens - The eating routine that limits fat and frequently soaked fat and cholesterol. They help in lessening the danger of coronary illness and corpulence.

Lyme illness - It is otherwise called Lyme borreliosis. It is a bacterial (Borrelia type) disease spread to people by contaminated ticks of the Ixodes family. A few people with Lyme sickness experience influenza like side effects in the beginning periods, for example, weakness, muscle torment, joint agony, migraines, fever, chills and neck solidness. Later manifestations incorporate issues influencing the sensory system and heart.

Melancholy – Depression (significant burdensome issue or clinical discouragement) is a typical however genuine state of mind issue. It causes serious manifestations that influence how you feel, think, and handle every day exercises, for example, resting, eating, or working.

To be determined to have despondency, the indications must be available for in any event two weeks.

Mumps - It is an infectious malady brought about by the mumps infection that goes starting with one individual then onto the next through salivation, nasal emissions, and close to home contact. It is otherwise called plague parotitis. Indications of mumps typically show up inside about fourteen days of introduction to the infection. Influenza like indications might be the first to show up, including weariness, body hurts, cerebral pain, loss of hunger and poor quality fever.

Nephron - It is gotten from the Greek word, 'nephros' signifying "kidney". It is the essential auxiliary and utilitarian unit of the kidney. The fundamental capacity is to expel abundance water, squanders and different substances from blood and return substances like sodium, potassium or phosphorus at whatever point any of these substances run low in the human body.

Nephropathy – It is otherwise called kidney sickness or renal infection. It is harm to or ailment of a kidney. Nephritis is a fiery kidney sickness. Nephrosis is noninflammatory nephropathy. Diabetic nephropathy is harm to kidneys brought about by diabetes.

Nerve center - It is an area of the cerebrum answerable for the creation of a considerable lot of the body's basic hormones, compound substances that help control various cells and organs. This region of the cerebrum houses the pituitary organ and different organs in the body.

Neuron - It is otherwise called a neuron or nerve cell. It is the fundamental structure square of the sensory system. Neurons are like different cells in the human body in various ways, yet there is one key contrast among neurons and different cells. Neurons are particular to transmit data all through the body. These profoundly particular nerve cells are answerable for conveying data in both substance and electrical structures.

Neuropathy – It is utilized to depict an issue with the nerves, for the most part the 'fringe nerves' instead of the 'focal sensory system' (the cerebrum and spinal line). The term 'neuropathy' covers a wide region and numerous nerves, however the issue it causes relies upon the kind of nerves that are influenced in particular tangible nerves, engine nerves and autonomic nerves. Mononeuropathy alludes to a solitary nerve being influenced. Polyneuropathy implies a few nerves are influenced.

NIDDM - It is Non-Insulin Dependent Diabetes Mellitus, a type of diabetes where insulin generation is lacking or the body has gotten impervious to insulin. It is otherwise called Type 2 diabetes. Normal side effects incorporate expanded thirst, expanded craving, visit pee, feeling worn out and unexplained weight reduction.

OGTT - It is the Oral Glucose Tolerance Test. Right now, standard portion of glucose is ingested by mouth and blood levels are checked two hours after the fact. It very well may be utilized to analyze prediabetes and diabetes. An OGTT is most regularly done to check for diabetes that happens with pregnancy (gestational diabetes).

Osteoporosis (diminishing bones) – The word osteoporosis is from the Greek expressions for "permeable bones". It is an ailment where the bones become delicate from loss of tissue, commonly because of hormonal changes or lack of Calcium or Vitamin D. Side effects incorporate spinal pain, slow loss of stature with stooped stance and crack of the spine, wrist or hip.

Pad (Peripheral Arterial Disease) – It is a narrowing of the periphery passages to the legs, stomach, arms and head - most usually in the stockpile courses of the legs. Pad resembles Coronary Artery Disease (CAD). Both PAD and CAD are brought about by atherosclerosis that strait and squares supply routes in different basic districts of the body. The most well-known side effect of PAD in the lower furthest points is an agonizing muscle squeezing in the hips, thighs or calves when strolling, climbing stairs or working out.

Pancreas - It is a glandular organ in the stomach related framework and endocrine arrangement of vertebrates. In individuals, it is arranged in the stomach gap behind the stomach. It is around 6 inches in length. It is an endocrine organ creating a few significant hormones. It is additionally a stomach related organ discharging pancreatic juice containing stomach related catalysts.

Parkinson's ailment – It is otherwise called idiopathic or essential parkinsonism, hypokinetic unbending disorder. It is a degenerative issue of the focal sensory system predominantly influencing the engine framework. This malady influences development, autonomic brokenness, neuropsychiatric issues (state of mind, cognizance, conduct or thought changes), and tangible and rest challenges.

Phenylketonuria (PKU) - It is an acquired issue that expands the degrees of a substance called phenylalanine in the blood. On the off chance that PKU isn't dealt with, phenylalanine can develop to hurtful levels in the body, causing scholarly inability and different genuine medical issues. Phenylalanine is a structure square of proteins (an amino corrosive) that is acquired through the eating regimen. It is found in all proteins and in some fake sugars.The most extreme type of this issue is known as exemplary PKU. Newborn children with great PKU seem typical until they are a couple of months old. Without treatment, these youngsters build up a changeless scholarly handicap. Seizures, deferred advancement, conduct issues, and mental issue are additionally normal. Less extreme types of this condition, in some cases called variation PKU and non-PKU hyperphenylalaninemia, have a little danger of cerebrum harm. Individuals with mellow cases may not require treatment with a low-phenylalanine diet.

Phlebotomy – It is the withdrawal of blood from the arm veins.

Polycystic ovary disorder (PCOS) - It is otherwise called Stein-Leventhal disorder. It is a lot of indications because of raised male hormones in ladies. Signs and side effects of PCOS incorporate unpredictable or no menstrual periods, substantial periods, abundance body and facial hair, skin break out and pelvic torment. Related conditions incorporate sort 2 diabetes, heftiness, coronary illness and endometrial malignant growth.

Polydipsia - It is gotten from the Greek word, 'polys' signifies "without a doubt" or "many" and 'dipsa' signifies "thirst". It is the term given to over the top thirst and is one of the underlying side effects of both diabetes mellitus and diabetes insipidus. It is additionally typically joined by brief or delayed dryness of the mouth. A portion of the causes are looseness of the bowels, regurgitating, bountiful perspiring, noteworthy blood misfortune and so forth.

Polyphagia - It is gotten from the Greek word, 'polys' signifies "without a doubt" or "many" and 'phago' signifies "eating". It is the term used to depict over the top craving or expanded hunger and is one of the three fundamental indications of diabetes. It is here and there known as hyperphagia. It generally happens from the get-go over the span of diabetic ketoacidosis.

Polyuria - It is a condition normally characterized as the generation of strangely enormous volumes of weaken pee. Expanded creation and entry of pee may likewise be named diuresis. The most widely recognized reason for polyuria in the two grown-ups and youngsters is uncontrolled diabetes mellitus which causes osmotic diuresis.

Protein - They are huge biomolecules or macromolecules. They are polymer chains made of amino acids connected together by peptide bonds. During human absorption, proteins are separated in the stomach to littler peptide chains by means of hydrochloric corrosive and protease activities. They are fundamental supplements for the human body. They are one of the structure squares of body tissue.

Psoriasis - It is an immune system ailment portrayed by patches of irregular skin which are regularly red, irritated and textured. It is portrayed by skin cells that increase up to multiple times quicker than ordinary. It happens on the knees, elbows and scalp and it can likewise influence the middle, palms and bottoms of the feet. The primary kinds of psoriasis are plaque, guttate, converse, pustular and erythrodermic.

Pubescence - National Institute of Child Health and Human Development characterizes Puberty is the time in life when a kid or young lady turns out to be explicitly full grown. It is a procedure that generally occurs between ages 10 and 14 for young ladies and ages 12 and 16 for young men. It causes physical changes and impacts youngsters and youngsters in a sudden manner. In young ladies: bosom improvement; hair development in pubic region and armpits; monthly cycle occurs finally. In young men: Testicles and penis getting greater; h

Queasiness - It is the vibe of an inclination to upchuck. Sickness can be intense and brief, or it tends to be drawn out. At the point when drawn out, it is a weakening manifestation. Sickness (and heaving) can be mental or physical in starting point. It can begin from issues in the cerebrum or organs of the upper gastrointestinal tract. It likewise might be brought about by maladies of numerous organs outside of the gastrointestinal framework.

RBG/CBG - It is Random Blood Glucose or Casual Blood Glucose test. It is a glucose test taken from a non-fasting subject. This test expect an ongoing dinner and in this way has a higher reference an incentive than the fasting glucose test. As per American Diabetes Association (ADA), the reference esteems for a "typical" irregular glucose test in a normal grown-up are 79 - 140 mg/dl (4.4 - 7.8 mmol/l), between 140 - 200 mg/dl is considered pre-diabetes or more 200 mg/dl is viewed as diabetes.

Removal - It is the evacuation of an appendage by injury, medicinal ailment or medical procedure. As a careful measure, it is utilized to control torment or an illness procedure in the influenced appendage, for example, harm or gangrene.

Retinopathy – It is industrious or intense harm to the retina of the eye. Every now and again, it is a visual appearance of foundational malady as found in diabetes or hypertension. Retinopathy that is caused because of diabetes mellitus and blood vessel hypertension is named as diabetic retinopathy and hypertensive retinopathy individually. All types of diabetic eye sickness can possibly cause serious vision misfortune and visual deficiency.

Rheumatoid joint inflammation (RA) - It is an immune system malady that can cause constant irritation of the joints and different regions of the body. Manifestations and signs remember joint torment for the feet, hands and knees; swollen joints; fever; delicate joints; loss of joint capacity; firm joints; weariness; joint disfigurement. In RA, different joints are generally, yet not constantly, influenced in an even example. 80% of RA patients have "rheumatoid factor", an immunizer that can be found in the blood.

Rubella - It is an intense, infectious viral disease brought about by the rubella infection. It is otherwise called German measles or three-day measles. While the ailment is commonly mellow in youngsters, it has genuine outcomes in pregnant ladies causing fetal demise or inherent imperfections known as innate rubella disorder (CRS). The rubella infection is transmitted via airborne beads when tainted individuals wheeze or hack. People are the main known host. There is no particular treatment for rubella however the sickness is preventable by immunization (rubella antibody).

SMBG - It is Self - Monitoring of Blood Glucose. It is a significant part of present day treatment for diabetes mellitus. SMBG has been suggested for individuals with diabetes and their medicinal services experts so as to accomplish a particular degree of glycemic control and to forestall hypoglycemia. By observing blood glucose without anyone else's input, can ready to make changes to their nourishment or potentially practice on the off chance that they have a test outcome that is excessively low or high. Making these little changes will assist them with remaining on target, rest easy thinking about their diabetes, and it can likewise bring down the danger of creating medical issues after some time. Model - Person utilizing numerous day by day infusions of insulin (≥ 4 times each day) or utilizing an insulin siphon, at that point SMBG ought to be ≥ 4 times each day.

Stroke – It is a condition wherein blood supply to be the cerebrum is influenced. A stroke can some of the time lead to changeless harm including correspondence issues, loss of motion and visual issues. Factually, individuals with diabetes have a higher danger of biting the dust from coronary illness and stroke than the all inclusive community. The two principle types are (1) Ischaemic – where a blood coagulation shapes in the cerebrum. (2) Haemorrhagic - whereby a vein in the cerebrum blasts and causes a mind drain.

Sugar - Any nourishment that is especially wealthy in the intricate sugar starch, (for example, grains, bread and pasta) or straightforward carbs, for example, sugar (found in treats, jams and sweets). It is a natural particle comprising of carbon, hydrogen and oxygen iotas, as a rule with a hydrogen-oxygen molecule proportion of 2:1 (as in water).

Sulfonylurea - They are a class of natural mixes utilized in medication and horticulture. They are antidiabetic medicates that are utilized in the administration of diabetes mellitus type 2. Their principle work is to expand insulin discharge from the beta cells in the pancreas.

Swelling – Any strange general expanding or increment in distance across of the stomach zone. The side effect related with swelling is an impression that the stomach area is full or extended. It might cause stomach agony or brevity of breath.

Tamoxifen - It is a drug that is utilized to forestall bosom disease in ladies and treat bosom malignant growth in ladies and men. It is accessible as a nonexclusive drug. It obstructs the activity of estrogen, a female hormone and specific kinds of bosom malignant growth expect estrogen to develop.

Tumor - They are a gathering of anomalous cells that structure protuberances or developments. Various kinds of tumors develop and carry on in an unexpected way, contingent upon whether they are non-harmful (amiable) or pre-carcinogenic (pre-threatening) or (dangerous). It is otherwise called a neoplasm.

Type 2 Polyglandular immune system disorder (PGA II) - It is the most well-known of the immunoendocrinopathy disorders. It comprises of Addison infection in addition to either an immune system thyroid sickness or type 1 diabetes mellitus related with hypogonadism, malignant pallor, celiac illness, and ongoing essential biliary cirrhosis.

Ulcers – It is a sore, which implies it's an open, difficult injury. Normal types of ulcers are peptic ulcer, mouth ulcer, corneal ulcer, a venous ulcer, stress ulcer, pressure ulcers, genital ulcer, diabetic foot ulcer, and so forth., Peptic ulcers are in reality extremely normal.

Uneasiness – A sentiment of stress and apprehension. General indications incorporate sentiments of frenzy, dread; cold or sweat-soaked hands or feet; brevity of breath; dry mouth; heart palpitations; queasiness; tipsiness, and so on.,

Vasopressin - It is otherwise called antidiuretic hormone (ADH). It is a neurohypophysial hormone found in many well evolved creatures. In many species it contains arginine and in this way it is called Arginine Vasopressin (AVP) or Argipressin. It is a pituitary hormone that demonstrations to advance the maintenance of water by the kidneys and increment pulse.

Vasopressinase - During pregnancy, ladies produce vasopressinase in the placenta, which separates antidiuretic hormone (ADH). Gestational Diabetes Insipidus is thought to happen with over the top generation and/or debilitated freedom of vasopressinase.

Waterfalls – It is a blurring of the focal point in the eye prompting a lessening in a dream. It can influence one or the two eyes. Side effects may incorporate blurred hues, foggy vision, coronas around light, issue with splendid lights and inconvenience seeing around evening time.

Weariness - Extreme tiredness coming about because of mental or physical effort or disease. It is an ordinary aftereffect of working, mental pressure, overstimulation, under-incitement, gloom, absence of rest. Different causes may likewise incorporate harming or nutrient or mineral inadequacies.

Weight - A turmoil including inordinate muscle versus fat that expands the danger of medical issues. Stoutness is most ordinarily brought about by a mix of over the top nourishment consumption, absence of physical movement and hereditary helplessness. It is a main preventable reason for death around the world, with expanding rates in grown-ups and youngsters. Changes to eat less and practicing are the fundamental medicines.

Wilson's ailment - It is otherwise called Wilson infection or hepatolenticular degeneration. It is an uncommon acquired issue that makes a lot of copper gather in the liver, mind and other indispensable organs. Indications regularly start between the ages of 12 and 23. In an ordinary individual, copper is retained from nourishment and any abundance is discharged through bile (a substance delivered in the liver). Be that as it may, in individuals with Wilson's infection, copper isn't disposed of appropriately and rather gathers, potentially to a dangerous level. It very well may be treated with medicine.

Youthfulness - It is gotten from the Latin word "adolescere" which signifies "to grow up". It is the period following the beginning of pubescence during which a youngster forms from a kid into a grown-up.

26. REFERENCES

http://www.joslin.org/info/what_is_insulin_resistance.html.AccessedApril28,2014. Joslin Diabetes Center.

http://www.joslin.org/info/insulin_a_to_z_a_guide_on_different_types_of_insulin.html. AccessedApril28,

http://link.springer.com/article/10.1007%2Fs00428-004-1021-5

http://medical-dictionary.thefreedictionary.com/biofeedback

http://pancreas.org/patients/cystic-fibrosis/

http://timesofindia.indiatimes.com/15-home-remedies-to-treat-diabetes-heart ailments/articleshow/20240984.cms

http://www.aboutdiabetesinformation.com/diabetesurinetest-benedicts-test.php

http://www.acupuncturetoday.com/archives2003/nov/11lo.html

http://www.antibodies-online.com/kit/504750/T3,+T4++TSH+CLIA+Kit/

http://www.biothesiometer.com/

http://www.diabetes.co.uk/alternative-treatment/Chinese-medicine-acupuncture-diabetes.html

http://www.diabetes.co.uk/alternative-treatment/Diabetes-and-Aromatherapy.html

http://www.diabetes.co.uk/alternative-treatment/Diabetes-and-Ayurverdic-medicine.html

http://www.diabetes.co.uk/alternative-treatment/Diabetes-and-Biofeedback.html

http://www.diabetes.co.uk/alternative-treatment/Diabetes-and-Massage-Therapy-Reflexology.html

American Diabetes Association. Living with Diabetes: Insulin Basics. June 7, 2013. http://www.diabetes.org/living-with-diabetes/treatment-and-care/medication/insulin/insulin-basics.html. Accessed April 28, 2014.

Joslin Diabetes Center. Managing Diabetes: What is Insulin Resistance? http://www.joslin.org/info/what_is_insulin_resistance.html. Accessed April 28, 2014.

Joslin Diabetes Center. Managing Diabetes: Insulin A to Z: A Guide on Different Types of Insulin.

http://www.joslin.org/info/insulin_a_to_z_a_guide_on_different_types_of_insulin.html.

Accessed April 28, 2014.

Mayo Clinic. Diabetes treatment: Using insulin to manage blood sugar. August 7, 2013. http://www.mayoclinic.org/diseases-conditions/diabetes/in-depth/diabetes-treatment/art-20044084. Accessed April 28, 2014.

http://www.diabetes.co.uk/Diabetes-herbal.html

http://www.diabetes.co.uk/emotions/diabetes-and-mindfulness.html

http://www.diabetes.co.uk/hemochromatotis-bronze-diabetes.html

http://www.diabetes.co.uk/insulin/Insulin-pumps.html

http://www.diabetes.co.uk/yoga-and-diabetes.html

http://www.diabetes.org/diabetes-basics/a-day-in-the-life-of-diabetes/

http://www.diabetes.org/diabetes-basics/common-terms/

http://www.diabetes.org/diabetes-basics/famous-people-working-to-stop-diabetes.html

http://www.diabetes.org/diabetes-basics/genetics-of-diabetes.html

http://www.diabetes.org/diabetes-basics/myths/

http://www.diabeteshealth.com/the-history-of-diabetes/

http://www.diabetesincontrol.com/diabetes-mellitus-and-infectious-diseases-controlling-chronic-hyperglycemia/

http://www.diabetesselfmanagement.com/diabetes-resources/definitions/biofeedback/

http://www.healthline.com/health/doppler-ultrasound-exam-of-an-arm-or-leg#Results5

http://www.homeveda.com/Natural-Remedies/Diabetes/Natural-Ayurvedic-Home-Remedies-for-Diabetes

http://www.indianmedicinalplants.info/articles/TEST-FOR-ACETONE-BODIES.html

http://www.joslin.org/info/oral_diabetes_medications_summary_chart.html

http://www.kodymedical.com/neuropathy.html

http://www.mayoclinic.org/diseases-conditions/peripheral-artery-disease/symptoms-causes/dxc-20167421

http://www.medical-library.net/content/view/1538/41/

http://www.medicalnewstoday.com/articles/7504.php

http://www.medicine.mcgill.ca/physio/vlab/bloodlab/mcv-mchc_n.htm

http://www.ncbi.nlm.nih.gov/pmc/articles/PMC3354930/table/T1/

http://www.ncbi.nlm.nih.gov/pubmed/759015

http://www.niddk.nih.gov/health-information/health-topics/diagnostic-tests/a1c-test-diabetes/Pages/index.aspx

http://www.radiologyinfo.org/en/info.cfm?pg=chestrad

http://www.radiologymasterclass.co.uk/tutorials/chest/chest_pathology/chest_pathology_start

http://www.theayurveda.org/ayurveda/natural-herbs-to-cure-diabetes-ailment/

http://www.webmd.com/diabetes/types-of-diabetes-mellitus

http://www.yogapoint.com/therapy/diabetes_yoga.htm

https://books.google.co.in/books?isbn=0070617678

https://en.wikipedia.org/wiki/Cirrhosis

https://en.wikipedia.org/wiki/Diabetes_insipidus

https://en.wikipedia.org/wiki/Diabetes_mellitus

https://en.wikipedia.org/wiki/Fibrosis

https://en.wikipedia.org/wiki/Glucose_test

https://en.wikipedia.org/wiki/History_of_diabetes

https://en.wikipedia.org/wiki/Mean_corpuscular_volume

https://en.wikipedia.org/wiki/Random_glucose_test

https://en.wikipedia.org/wiki/Urine_test_strip

https://labtestsonline.org/understanding/analytes/platelet/platelet-count/

https://labtestsonline.org/understanding/analytes/wbc/white-blood-cell-count/

https://medlineplus.gov/ency/article/000286.htm

https://medlineplus.gov/ency/article/003569.htm

https://medlineplus.gov/ency/article/003775.htm

https://medlineplus.gov/ency/article/003777.htm

https://medlineplus.gov/ency/article/003878.htm

https://nisargopcharashram.org/

https://taniloy.wordpress.com/2013/11/24/procedure-of-rotheras-test-for-ketone-bodies/

https://www.google.co.in/?gfe_rd=cr&ei=hYsRVrCdl7Dv8weFiITYCw#q=bronze+diabetes

https://www.ottawaheart.ca/test-procedure/treadmill-exercise-stress-test

https://www.tekscan.com/application-group/embedded-sensing/foot-mapping?tab=overview

https://www.vitamindcouncil.org/about-vitamin-d/testing-for-vitamin-d/

http://www.diabetes.ca/diabetes-and-you/what/history/

http://www.ncbi.nlm.nih.gov/pubmed/11953758

http://www.japi.org/special_issue_april_2011/01_Diabetic_History.pdf

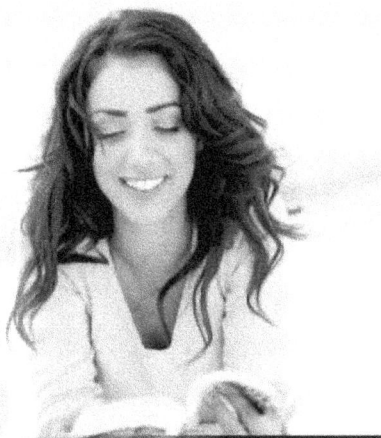

www.ingramcontent.com/pod-product-compliance
Lightning Source LLC
Chambersburg PA
CBHW021046210326
41598CB00016B/1108